Coming to Grief

Coming to Grief

A Survival Guide to Grief and Loss

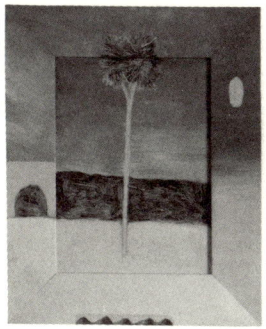

Pam Heaney

Longacre Press

ISBN 1 877135 64 X

First published by Longacre Press 2002
9 Dowling Street, Dunedin, New Zealand.

Book and cover design by Christine Buess
Printed by Brebner Print Ltd, Auckland, New Zealand

contents

This book is dedicated to
Jon-Luke
James
Damien
Jarred
Natasha

*You each are a note in the love song
of creation;
the harmony always is true.*

introduction

In a way this all began when I was driving buses. Nearly twenty years ago now. At least, that's when I became acutely aware of death. Yet I suspect my learning about grief began long before then – indeed when I look back I see that my whole life has been learning about how we grieve.

Twenty years ago, I was heading home one evening after completing the sight-seeing run. It was late, dark and cold; good enough reason to have fish and chips for tea. I was standing in the shop, having just given my order, when I heard an almighty thump from outside. 'An accident,' I thought. 'Someone has hit something.' Along with several others I rushed out to see what had happened. There was a body lying in the middle of the road.

I responded magnificently. Nobody could have wished for a better Manager of Operations. 'Come here', 'Go there', 'Ring for this', 'Ring for that', 'Stay with them', 'Look after those', 'Redirect here/there', 'Stop that'. Brilliant!

Yet I became increasingly aware that I could not go anywhere near the man who was lying in the middle of the road. And I didn't understand why that was so. He was lying on his back, his arms and legs spread-eagled. His head was turned to one side and his eyes were closed. There was (to me) no visible sign of injury, and perhaps most surprisingly, there was no blood. So why couldn't I move forward and attend to him? After all, I had my St John's Certificate and thought I was Superwoman – so why was I unable to render first aid? I organised everyone and everything with gusto and remember feeling somewhat guilty as I stood there, unable to move. My feet felt nailed to the ground.

But what I had started to realise was that I did not know, could not tell, whether this man was alive or dead. I could not recognise dead. Here I was, 34 years of age, and I did not know what death was.

The ambulance arrived, the man was carried away, and the crowd began to disperse. I approached the ambulance personnel and asked whether the person was alive. I was dismissed with a curt response, something along the lines that such information could not be revealed, and who the hell was I to ask such a thing anyway? So now not only was I still ignorant, but I was also hurt at being so dismissed. It all added to the shock.

I went home and had my fish and chips. Very soon afterward I promptly lost them. I was in shock all right!

The question of whether the man had been alive or dead remained with me, and the realisation that I didn't know how to recognise death nagged at me constantly. I bought the papers until I read a brief report of the accident. Eyewitnesses reported seeing a man being struck by a car that threw him into the air and then into the path of another. The second was unable to stop, and it had run over him. He had died as the result of his injuries. I read his funeral notice.

Distressing as all this was, it still didn't tell me whether he had been dead or alive at the scene of the accident.

For the first time, I seriously began to think about life and death, and realised that death was something that would ultimately happen to me. I was still rather bemused by the fact that I couldn't recognise 'dead'. Until one day the thought presented itself to me as 'If I don't know what dead is, maybe I don't know what alive is either'.

This realisation provoked a serious line of thought. This was the start of my journey into grief. It was as if this single event had turned me upside down and shaken me apart. There began a process of looking at my own existence and deciding if I was truly alive. Did I pass each day in a monotonous routine that had little meaning or purpose? Was I living my life as I wanted to? Or was I always striving to make someone else happy and meet their expectations of me? Was I able to express myself creatively, spontaneously, and feel all there was to feel, be it joy, pleasure, sadness, rage or love? In short, the answers were yes, no, yes and no. At that point I decided I was therefore more dead than alive.

I then began the process of looking at life and death; and of looking at myself in relation to this. Those aspects of my life that are no longer appropriate I have discarded, those that are inadequate and damaged I am healing, and those that have been absent I am developing. The whole is being put back together in a new way that is an honest reflection of me and my desire to be fully alive. Now – rather than deny, avoid or try to control difficult and painful issues – I am learning to be self-aware, and to base my self-esteem and self-acceptance on personal responsibility (rather than on the management of crisis or by trying to be Superwoman).

My journey has taken me into Funeral Directing. I still find it ironic that I learnt so much about life and living by dealing with death and dying. It has led me to university, and to complete other studies to consolidate my practical experience. Along the way I have co-founded the Grief Education Trust, and helped initiate the National Association for Loss and Grief. I have conducted and promoted the importance of Critical Incident Stress Debriefing for people after traumatic events (such as the accident I witnessed), and I have worked with the dying and bereaved in an endless variety of situations. I have lectured in a wide range of tertiary institutions and directed educational programmes for health care professionals, volunteers, support groups, families and organisations. Through counselling, therapeutic workshops and grief recovery groups I have assisted people to move back into life after the dislocation of major loss.

I well remember when I had to ask myself why I was so passionately involved with grief, and to acknowledge just how much I enjoyed the work I was doing. My answer nowadays is the same as it was then. In giving others permission to grieve, I am in essence giving myself permission to do so as well. And I can now acknowledge that I had much in my life to grieve about. My study of grief continues, on both a personal and professional level.

There is also another dimension that fuels my ongoing

involvement in this work. Grieving is something we all have to learn at some stage, but this learning process is not voluntary and is often not recognised in Western, Pakeha culture. Grieving is often resisted by many of us and the social norms that people have developed in order to cope have their foundation in myths. Consequently many people carry large amounts of long-standing unresolved grief. My experience has revealed that this affects their health, spiritual well-being and their ability to function, both at work and in relationships, in ways that are life-enhancing and which provide any degree of satisfaction. The personal and social costs of this unresolved grief are enormous, but again largely not understood.

This book is my attempt to assist those who genuinely seek to learn about grief, and to change the current cultural attitudes by challenging the social myths that give rise to them. These social myths do little more than force people to be stoic about their grief, and they offer nothing to assist its resolution.

Much has been written about grief and grieving, but most of the material falls into one of two categories. The first is academic and for the average person, makes heavy reading (especially if they are in the middle of grieving). The second category describes personal experiences: telling of events in someone else's life and how they responded to it. Both can be helpful if your experience relates to the material, although it is disconcerting and disorientating if it does not. Neither category moves beyond the descriptive.

Hence this book. I don't just want you to learn about the general phenomen of grief or about how someone else has grieved. Instead I want you to come to know your own grief, when it is happening, what it is about and how to resolve it in a way that is appropriate for you. I want to offer something effective and honest. 'Time will heal' is one of the many lies that keeps people trapped in their grief, sometimes for a lifetime. I don't want that to happen to you. Not if you want to be fully alive.

So here are ten of the most commonly used and accepted myths regularly found in my work. I set about to counter each by looking at why we grieve, what grief is and how it affects us, why everyone does their grieving just a little bit differently from everyone else, and what we need to do in order to finish and move on from it. Included are a variety of exercises to help make the information personal to you. I have also put forward a few thoughts at the end of each chapter where I encourage you to pause and reflect. Ultimately you will realise that grieving is not about forgetting what has happened or 'letting go' of a loved one. Rather it is about reconstructing the relationship in a way that is now more appropriate, and integrating the experience so that you can live with both. It sounds simple. And it is. But it is not easy. And it is a process, not an event.

So take your time from here on. Read at your own pace, and be gentle with yourself as you do so. If you have a friend or someone special whom you trust and can share it with, it will make for easier travelling. My hope is that you will learn a good deal to help you along your way.

Pam Heaney
February, 2002

1 *Myth: You only grieve when someone dies.*

Reality: We grieve whenever we lose anything, whether it be someone or something.

Grief accompanies loss. Any loss. Big losses, personal losses, petty little not-worth-talking-about losses. We even grieve for those losses we only *think* might happen. Grief is our response to loss.

Grief is a natural emotion and our very normal response to a loss of any kind.

Admittedly in our Western culture we think that people only grieve when someone dies. They do grieve then, of course, but we think that's all there is to it. We are not taught about grief. Rather we learn about it from hearing the likes of the myth I've chosen as a chapter heading, or observing the maladjusted grieving responses of others. Consequently we do not understand what causes grief, how to recognise it when we (or another) is in the midst of it, or what to do about it in order to resolve it. As a nation and as a generation, we have lost the know-how of dealing with grief. We deny or are simply unaware of what we need to do in order to adjust to loss and the change this always brings.

To begin to appreciate the grieving process, we need to adjust our thinking. This requires a generosity on our part, both in regard to others, and towards ourselves. It also requires a willingness to be honest, take time and do some soul searching. Oops. All of a sudden things are sounding serious. Which is why this is about as far as most people get. They prefer instead to avoid or dismiss what is happening to them (or others) by regurgitating myths. Much easier. Far less time consuming. And it also means that any personal responsibility for dealing with the grief can be side-stepped. Again, much easier to blame something or someone else for what has happened or for how we are feeling.

But for those of you who are seeking more and who want to increase your awareness about grief and the grieving process, let us begin with changing our thinking.

If, as I've already stated, grief accompanies loss, we there-fore start by identifying losses. The majority of people focus on the immediate crisis or event that has just happened. And that's a good place to start. However, now we will move beyond that and ask ourselves what losses that person (or ourselves) might be experiencing as a result of that crisis or event.

Take redundancy for instance. The loss of a job is the obvi-ous and presenting loss. But as people who have experienced redundancy are aware, there are a number of other losses as well. How about this for starters:

There is the loss of
- Certainty • Life the way it used to be • Friends and colleagues • Income (or role of income earner) • Hopes and dreams • Financial security • Identity • Independence • Self-worth • Self-confidence • Structure and routine • Success • Pride • Sense of belonging • Control of your life • Opportunity • Social status • Peace of mind • Health

How each person experiences redundancy will be different, and unique to them, and so the losses involved will also be unique. But this list is a fair representation of what's involved. We don't usually think in terms of losses and we also don't realise the extent of what is going on for us. It's not just that 'I have been made redundant'. Rather it's 'This is what it means to me to have been made redundant – I have lost all these things'. No wonder we feel so awful. But what the heck! It's just a job. It's not as if I can be grieving, because nobody has died. And we're told that all we have to do is pull ourselves together and think positively. And still we feel awful. And don't know why.

Identifying losses has several purposes. Importantly, it legitimises our experience. It makes what has happened to us real and we are given the opportunity, permission and encouragement to tell it the way it is for us. Never mind how it might have been for anyone else, or what others might think. At last, we can begin to own what we have experienced but have never been allowed or were maybe too scared, to share. This is an important distinction to make. Identifying losses is not about blaming others, or criticising what was or wasn't done by someone else at the time of the loss. It is about admitting and owning what that experience was like for me.

And no, this is not being selfish.

In identifying our losses, we help ourselves enormously. In most cases, people do not understand why they feel the way they do. But when they begin to understand that grief is connected to loss and they can identify all the losses they are experiencing, then they gain some insight into why they are feeling the way they are.

This usually comes as a relief. When someone is experiencing grief over a death, or is grieving for any other loss, the effects are devastating and debilitating. And yet it is not like an illness or accident where the injury is apparent. There are no bandages or crutches or medical certificates to indicate to others that they are hurting, or that they have reason to be hurting. And because the hurt cannot be justified, it is rationalised instead. How often have you heard someone say 'It was only the cat (a holiday, an exam, a piece of jewellery) – I shouldn't be feeling like this.' And the bit that remains unspoken goes something like 'God, I must be stupid' or 'What's wrong with me?'

Several other things also become apparent when we begin to think 'losses' rather than 'event'. People begin to realise that they haven't just lost a job. They begin to understand and appreciate that many other things are also going on for them at the same time. Admittedly in any situation there is the obvious loss, but there are always more. When the losses are all identified (and this usually takes some time if it is done honestly and sincerely), it often happens that one of those subsequent or intrinsic losses is of more importance than the obvious loss.

Let me put it another way. We hear that someone's cat has died. For one person this may be no big deal. For another it may be an enormous relief that the cat has died. Maybe it was attacking the neighbour's hens. For another person it may be a time consuming and demanding exercise to explain to the children what has happened and to dispose of puss in a way that is acceptable to them. For the elderly person who has lived alone with their cat for many years, the death of their cat may represent the loss of being needed, the loss of unconditional love, and the loss of companionship. For many in this situation, it also frequently means the loss of a reason to continue living.

Only the person who is experiencing the loss can determine the importance of that loss. For them. It pays to listen very carefully to what someone tells us before we make our response. More often than not, people respond with what that loss would mean for themselves which is sometimes very little, rather than pausing to appreciate what the significance of the loss could mean to anyone else.

And it is a futile and useless exercise to try and compare losses or grief. There is only what my loss means to me, and what your loss means to you. Hence for one worker, redundancy may present the opposite of the picture I have painted and bring opportunity for change, retraining, the chance to alter their lifestyle or be free of something they have not enjoyed doing for a long time. Even so there will be losses involved, but of a less significant nature. And herein lies the difficulty in understanding the grief of another. We tend to interpret another's experience according to our own, or according to the prevalent societal expectation (or myth).

It is important to recognise that the same loss can mean different things to different people. Because the amount of grief that accompanies the loss usually equals the importance of the loss. Only I can determine that for me; only you can decide that for you. A general rule of thumb to remember is that the bigger (or more important) the loss is for us, the bigger (or more) grief we experience. They are relative to each other.

Loss is associated with all life changes in varying degrees. And when these life changes highlight a major loss it is appropriate that we acknowledge this and attend to the grief involved. Grief needs no invitation to come calling. It arrives. Loss activates grief as surely as night follows day. It is in our nature for this to happen; it is the way we adjust to change in our lives. Grief is what enables us to say goodbye when we don't want to say goodbye, be it to a person, a thing, or a part of our life.

Losses can be many and varied. Here is just one method that will help to recognise them.

Loss can be the result of:

Loss of Part of Self

Physical Loss

Either structurally – through the loss of a limb, organ, disfigurement.

Or through the loss of function – as stroke, paralysis, blindness, infertility.

Psychological Loss

For example: memory, judgement, pride, control, status, usefulness, independence, esteem, values, ideals, innocence, dignity.

Social Loss

For example: loss of social role, employment, opportunity to parent.

Loss also results from

Loss of External Objects
For example: possessions, money, property, pets, jewels.

Developmental Losses
Such as birth traumas, friends, opportunities, normality, childhood.

Fantasy Loss
Of our dreams, goals, expectations, wishes.

Loss of Significant Person
By death, separation, desertion, abortion, stillbirth, rejection, adoption.

Community and Cultural Losses
From immigration, urban renewal, refugee experience, disaster.

We can now begin to appreciate that losses come in all shapes and sizes. They can be personal, environmental, developmental, relational and natural. They can be external, about things and people, and they can be internal, about ourselves. It may, however, take some time to identify the particular loss which is most significant for us. But we need to grieve for every single one of them (to a greater or lesser degree) in order to dispel the sadness within us that results from our experience.

If we choose to believe in the myth that 'You only grieve when somebody dies', our losses go unrecognised, as does the fact that what we are experiencing is grief. We do not recognise it for ourselves, and neither do others recognise it in us. Conversely we do not recognise the grief that others may be experiencing. This is known as disenfranchised grief. And because it is not understood, it is repressed. And grief that is continually repressed becomes chronic depression.

When we move beyond this myth and allow ourselves to acknowledge our losses and natural grief response, we move toward health and healing.

Food For Thought

Here are some typical life scenarios. Take time now to reflect on them with new awareness and consider thoughtfully what each might render in terms of loss for the person involved. Refer to the earlier lists to assist you, but also be creative and list your own ideas. You are now making a loss profile.

- A four-year-old returns home from playschool to find the door to her rabbit hutch open and her pet gone. She would have told Grandad, who used to live next door, but she has been told that he has gone on a long holiday. But Grandad has not written her a letter, nor sent her a postcard nor even telephoned her, and they always used to write letters to each other. Nobody at home will even talk to her about Grandad.
  What are the losses for the four-year-old?

- A 15-year-old is causing concern at school. Her grades have unaccountably slipped; she has become moody, withdrawn and often aggressive – not like her at all. Her

Grandad died six months ago, and her Nanna is now coming to live with her family. Nanna will sleep in what was her bedroom, and the 15-year-old will now sleep in the caravan in the back yard.
What are the losses for the 15-year-old?

- At 22 he is on his first overseas trip and breaks his leg while skiing in China. He is in a 24-bed hospital ward and will be in traction there for six months.
What are the losses for the 22 year old?

- At 35 years of age she is married with four children and is pregnant again. The most recent scan caused concern and further tests reveal the child she is carrying has spina bifida. She and her husband decide to have an abortion.
What are the losses for the 35-year-old?

- An 11-year-old lives with his mother in the South Island. He is unhappy at school and his behaviour is becoming aggressive and troublesome. His parents separated last year and his father now has a new partner and has shifted to a town in the North Island.
What are the losses for the 11-year-old?

- She is 64 years of age and lives with her husband who retired two years ago. She has just been informed that her son has been made a director of the company that employed her husband for 35 years.
What are the losses for the 64-year-old?

Personal Loss Profile

The previous material will hopefully have helped you to think about your own experiences (and consequently yourself) in a different way. So here is an opportunity for you to reconsider a specific experience or event that is important for you.

The event I choose to reflect on is:

These are the losses I experienced when this happened:

Summary of Key Points

- Grief is our natural, normal response to a loss of any kind.

- Altering our thinking to consider losses (rather than focusing solely on the event) is the first step to understanding grief.

- Completing a Loss Profile is a helpful way of identifying our losses. (Completing a Loss Profile when someone else is grieving can also be the first step to our understanding their grief.)

- There is never only one loss. There is the obvious or presenting loss of someone or something, and also our personal losses as the result of this.

- The significance of any loss can only be determined by the person who is experiencing that loss.

- The amount of the grief experienced will usually equal the amount of significance we attach to that loss.

- The losses and subsequent grief of one person cannot be compared with the losses and grief of any other person – even when the losses appear to be of a similar nature.

2 *Myth: Just focus on the positives and you'll be right.*

Reality: When a loss occurs, there are always two things going on. Both need to be attended to.

It's about here that people begin to say 'Yes, but…! There are always the positive aspects to focus on. Think of the good things you have.' And I would never deny that. However there are two things going on when there is loss and both need to be dealt with separately. There are the positives, or gains that ultimately result from the loss AND there are the losses. In our society we are apt to focus on the positives or the 'nice' things and not bother with the losses. 'If I try harder, do it better, think more positively, keep smiling, it *should* be all right.' And then we wonder what is wrong with us when things don't get better or come right, and we still feel awful. Unfortunately, the positives do not cancel out the losses and no matter how hard we focus on the good of any situation, it will never make the 'bad' go away.

What happens all too frequently is that the separate losses and gains become mixed up together and people feel confused. They begin to feel inadequate or guilty, and sometimes as if they are going mad. Their reasoning is (and others are quick to tell them this) that they should be happy because they have so many positive things to enjoy. The reality is that they often feel flat, sad and confused, and yet if life is supposedly so good, they ask themselves, why should they? It makes no sense. 'I shouldn't be feeling this way. I must be selfish and ungrateful.'

Let's take a 'for instance'. There is the case of parents who have, quite naturally, looked forward to the birth of a healthy, normal child, but whose expectations have not been met. Instead they have a child who has spina bifida or Down's syndrome or some other impairment. There is often little time afforded these parents in which to adjust their expectations and acknowledge the multitude of confusing feelings that accompany this new reality. Most often they are expected to immediately accept, love and care for this little piece of humanity that is entirely dependent on them. And amazingly they do. There are the positive feelings that are related to being a parent, having created this miracle, their child being alive, and the loving and pleasure that brings in its own right. There are also the so-called negative feelings that are related to unfulfilled hopes, new and now different responsibilities, the fact that their child is not like everyone else's and the subsequent ongoing losses that result from this. But rarely are these feelings acknowledged or perceived as legitimate, and what is even more rare, is that parents should be allowed to have them, let alone express them and grieve. How many have felt disappointment, however fleeting, when the birth of a child revealed the gender to be other than the gender hoped for? And then felt guilty for having had this feeling? Feeling disappointed does not mean that you are a bad parent or were wrong to have had this feeling. It does mean that for a moment you were disappointed when you lost your expectation, and possibly, future dreams. Then followed a process (however transient or drawn out) during which you were able to adjust to the new reality and lovingly embrace your child.

There are always two things going on when people have accidents or illnesses that leave them with different abilities. All the positives are accentuated – lucky to be alive, can still do this (whatever 'this' is), lots of people are worse off than they are. But the frustration and disappointment of now not being able to play football or practise ballet, of having lost life the way it was, of now being unable to do what they had always planned to do, largely go unaddressed. And when someone does take a risk and expresses their so-called negative feelings, suddenly support disappears and they are labelled as ungrateful or selfish.

There is the case of abortion. Just because someone elects to have an abortion does not mean that they will not grieve or experience loss. The people concerned may experience immense sadness at the loss of life, the loss of potential and that a hope or wish is not being fulfilled. All of this holds true even though, whatever the circumstances, their choice has been made with the best intentions.

There are losses in any situation. The majority of people are simply unaware of this – or do not want to be. In a new marriage or partnership one would hope that the positives involved will always outweigh the losses. But there are some losses. The loss of total independence, life the way it has been, the freedom to make decisions without reference to a partner. Perhaps there is the loss of financial security, loss of time to see friends or team mates. There's even the loss of bedspace! (Hopefully that's a positive). But it is a change. You might even lose a quiet night's sleep by having to listen to your partner snore. Sometimes it's only simple, little losses that are involved, but unless and until we acknowledge them they begin to impinge on our life, our feelings and our general state of well-being. Many do not understand why, in this supposed state of bliss, they often feel 'flat'. And so they chastise themselves for feeling this way.

There is even loss attached to success, promotion and achieving our goals. In my own experience going to 'Varsity was always a dream for me. I never thought it would really happen. It was a bit like pie in the sky. But I did make it, as a 'mature' student. I thoroughly enjoyed the experience, finished with a respectable degree (after having failed School Certificate) and felt rather proud of myself and what I had achieved. But about six months later I went into a bit of a slump, and I couldn't figure out why. The future looked promising, I had no worries, I had been to University (the positives). But it occurred to me that what I was experiencing was very like grief. Could I be grieving? What had I lost, if anything? I settled down with pencil and paper and began to realise that I had indeed lost something. There was the routine and security and structure of the last three years; there were the friends I had made and the cups of coffee in the café over which we discussed just about everything (a real sense of belonging); there was also the loss of my dream (never mind that I had achieved it, I had lost it in the process and now had no pie in the sky); and there was the loss of some whom I had previously thought of as friends but who were now threatened by me. Or the knowledge I had acquired. Or the experience I had had. Or something. Whatever it was, it resulted in a change in our relationship. In the face of this list I had to admit there was reason enough for me to be grieving.

But wait, as the TV adverts say, there's more. It took me quite a while longer to appreciate what was the most significant loss of all. With success came the loss of a way of living. I could no longer label myself as a failure, or stupid, or opt out of discussions or situations by claiming they were beyond me. This was an enormous realisation. I was shattered by it. And I was very, very scared.

Few others appreciated my predicament and I got the message pretty quickly that 'I had nothing to worry about' and 'Good heavens, I shouldn't be feeling like that', and that 'I shouldn't keep thinking of the past'; in other words, focus on the positive. To be truthful I was worried. I did feel like that and I couldn't help but think of the past and the change I was faced with making. I also felt very alone because there were few who understood the significance of what was a metamorphosis for me. However in identifying what was happening I was ultimately able to face this new reality and move on.

It's worthwhile to listen to yourself when you feel flat, sad, and mixed up, because you could be responding to the losses you are experiencing. And this is the bit we are never taught how to deal with or are allowed to acknowledge socially. This is grief. And the first step to dealing with it is to identify and acknowledge the losses we are experiencing, as covered in the previous chapter. As explained, doing this is the first step to resolving our grief and thereby adjusting back into life.

If we don't do this, we never deal with the losses, nor do we deal with the feelings that accompany them. Rather we create ways for ourselves to live with both. I have learned over the years that people have many ways of doing this. They learn to live with the pain of their losses, and not let it show; they learn to suppress their pain and deny their feelings and live in their heads; they then learn to control their feelings with their thinking; they learn to adjust their lifestyle and avoid things and people who remind them of their pain and losses; they learn to control how, if, and when others might express their pain (so they won't be touched by it); and a lot of people just get sick. Because grief just doesn't go away – and time does not heal. As you will see, that is a myth also.

To focus solely on the positives and ignore the losses, and our feelings as a result, is to make like the proverbial ostrich. If we train ourselves to become unaware of the other side of the coin, it doesn't mean that it isn't happening. There is never a question of whether we will or won't experience grief. Rather the question is 'how'. And if we don't care for ourselves enough to acknowledge our losses and attend to our grief, it will wait around until we do.

Grief lodges itself in our bodies. Every system of our body is affected by the unresolved grief that we store. It depletes our immune system, upsets our digestive system, affects our nerves, strains our muscles and causes us to breath shallowly as our bodies live in an ongoing state of arousal to either fight or flee from this truth, this pain, these feelings which it is harbouring.

Facing this however, can be hard work. It requires time and energy, honesty and is a very painful process. These are the reasons most people avoid grieving or looking at other than the positives. Think about it. If something is going to cause us pain, our instincts tell us to give it a miss. And if hard work is involved – usually our approach is to find an easier or smarter way of doing it. Or to get someone else to do it for us. But no one else can do our grieving for us. And so we play Pollyanna instead and 'focus on the positives.'

So there appears to be a conflict here. On the one hand grief is a natural, normal thing for us to experience; and on the other we have an in-built mechanism that steers us away from it.

Two things to look at. Number one, there is no getting away from it. Until it is acknowledged, and dealt with, grief stays inside of us and does its own thing. And, it is cumulative. That means is just grows and grows as each new loss that we do not acknowledge adds more grief to what is already stored. (I imagine a squirrel storing away nuts.) This accounts for our sometimes quite unreasonable responses in situations – you know, when you want to express a quite righteous and appropriate anger in a controlled and constructive way and all of a sudden – hey presto! Where did that outburst come from?

It's like we went in to the storage cupboard inside ourselves for a little bit of anger (one nut), but instead tapped into all our stored grief that had not been dealt with. In other words, we emptied the whole pantry of nuts. And of course, as our little pile of grief grows and grows, it requires more and more energy to contain it, and not let it show, and to get on with life as if there was nothing wrong. And then we wonder why we always feel tired. Storing unresolved grief leads to chronic depression.

Secondly, we need to be aware that what we resist, persists. In other words, if we continue to avoid dealing with our grief, we will continue to encounter situations that remind us we still have it to deal with. To avoid this fate we need to move toward acceptance, and the first step in this process is to acknowledge fully what is happening for us. And when we find it difficult or painful or don't know how to do this, the support from a therapist, selected friend or other trusted person can be invaluable and of great assistance.

I am not suggesting that we forever and always become immersed in only looking at the losses. That would be equally as unhelpful as the present myth we are dispelling. As in all things, there is a balance that is healthy. Neither are we required to make value calls about our losses. We do not have to justify or moralise our losses. Just remember that there are always two things going on. It is good to focus on the positive aspects of any change and to do so to the fullest extent. And to also give equal attention and respect to the losses. By doing this you are honouring yourself, your reality and your grief, and in doing so, it will assist you toward good health and in your relations with others.

We do ourselves a disservice when we play Pollyanna and just focus on the positives. To play Pollyanna with someone else and thus prevent them from honouring the whole of their experience, is abusive.

Food For Thought

Here is a place for you to pause and consider the 'two things' which might be happening for you. This exercise will help identify your conflicting feelings, and what they relate to. You may also find it helpful to write down your thoughts and to see whether this helps you express your feelings, or to lock them away.

- Choose an event to reflect on (or continue working with the one that you chose earlier).

- List the feelings you are most aware of in relation to it.

- Now list them again, but divide them as indicated.

  Pleasant or Positive   Unpleasant or Negative
  (or acceptable)   (or unacceptable)

- Consider what losses trigger the feelings listed on the right.

- What are the messages you give yourself to control these feelings?

- Which feelings are you able to express, and which feelings do you not show?

- What are you afraid might happen if you did show them?

Personal Awareness Check

Our early experiences of loss leave us with messages, feelings, fears and attitudes that we carry throughout life. Although often unconscious, these early messages influence us in how we deal with loss. It is helpful, then, to recognise these messages and prevent them from controlling our present reactions. This way we can change our behaviour.

Think about and describe an important loss you have experienced. (You may choose to continue working with the one you selected earlier, or choose a new one.)

1. What happened?
2. When did it occur?
3. How were you advised to cope with the experience by significant people in your life?
4. Who were these people?
5. What were your reactions at the time to their advice?
6. What did you eventually do?
7. Think of your own feelings about this loss and the attitudes you maintain now. Write down these feelings and attitudes.
8. How has the advice you were given and your own thinking helped you to:
   - understand your own reaction to loss?
   - understand other people's reaction to loss?

Summary of Key Points

- Any life situation involves both gains and losses. Both need to be attended to.

- We often feel sad, flat, and confused when these gains and losses are mixed up together and not dealt with separately.

- Even when we actively choose a particular course of action, we will still experience loss and grief as a result of our decision.

- We cannot control grief by rationalising it, or by only thinking positive thoughts.

- When we just focus on the positives we develop ostrich type behaviour and ignore our losses and grief.

- Grief that is unacknowledged and therefore unresolved is stored in our bodies where it remains until attended to.

- This stored grief affects every system of our bodies.

- What we resist, persists.

- The effects of unresolved grief are cumulative. It ultimately affects our health, well-being and relations with others.

- To appreciate our experience, we need to focus on both sides of the coin.

- When we prevent either ourselves or someone else from experiencing both sides of the coin, our behaviour is abusive.

3 Myth: *Grief is only sadness.*

Reality: *Grief touches the whole of our being. It affects us physically, intellectually, emotionally and spiritually, and as a consequence it influences our behaviour.*

What people think of as grief and what grief actually is, are often two very different things. Unfortunately we don't usually discover this until we experience a major loss and find ourselves in the middle of a distressing, worrying and frightening situation. Usually people equate grief with sadness, and think they should be over it in about six months. And it's not too surprising that people think this way.

Grief has been a taboo subject in our society, and so many of us have not been adequately taught about it. It was not until the work of Dr Elizabeth Kubler-Ross was published in the early 1960s that our awareness of grief was raised and that regular and ongoing systematic research into the subject was then carried out.

Grief may be our natural, normal response to loss, but it can also be a devastating and debilitating experience. Grief is more than just sadness.

There are many well-researched, common, identifiable grief reactions. And they are all deemed to be 'normal'. I hasten to add that not everyone who is grieving will experience all these things. And some reactions can be associated with other ailments. Having said that, if you identify with any of the listed manifestations and they accompany a major loss, then you too can consider yourself to be 'normal'.

Physical Sensations:

• Knots in the stomach • Weakness in the muscles • Hollowness in the stomach • Over sensitivity to noise • Tightness in the chest • Breathlessness • Lack of energy • Aches and pains • Sore joints • Headaches • Constipation/Diarrhoea • Dry mouth

Experiencing any or all of these physical sensations will drain you of energy and often these symptoms are not recognised as part of grief. I always encourage people to visit their doctor and tell him or her what has happened in their life and what symptoms they are experiencing. There may not be a connection but an astute doctor will carry out some basic physical tests to establish well-being. It may be as simple as checking iron levels, but this in itself will be helpful. The hard work of grieving takes a lot of energy and we need to be in good health to do it.

Feelings:

• Sadness • Anger • Guilt and self-reproach • Anxiety • Loneliness • Fatigue • Helplessness • Shock • Freedom • Relief • Numbness • Inadequacy • Hurt • Yearning

The frightening thing about our feelings is that we have to feel them. It is not enough to sit and talk about them. Sometimes the intensity of our feelings will also be frightening.

Feelings are often considered to be messy, and many of us have not been taught to express them in a healthy, constructive way. In fact, many of us have survived a long time by not allowing them to surface or at least by not letting others see how we really feel. So when these awful feelings like anger or guilt come along, we don't know what to do with them. And they make us worried that others will know that we feel this way and somehow think less of us for it.

Our feelings are an uncomfortable part of grief, both because we experience them intensely and because there are so many to cope with. We feel dreadful because we may begin to be angry at the person who has died, or the thing we have lost, or perhaps because we have been left to deal with the bills, or kids, or simply because we are on our own.

We then try to control what we are feeling with our thinking. Internal messages begin to sound like 'I shouldn't say such awful things about someone who has just died,' and then 'I must be an awful person for feeling and thinking the things I do'. And often the final footnote is something like this: 'If people really knew what I was feeling they would think I am a dreadful person. They would not like me any more'. And of course, we have to rationalise our anger by saying it's our fault, because this isn't grief. Or so we think.

And so grief becomes even more frightening. We become isolated from those who might be able to help us, and from those we need. We cannot tell them how we feel, because we are taught to feel embarrassed about doing so from a very early age.

Another feeling that is difficult to own and share, and which is not often associated with grief, is relief. At first, it is not easy to see how relief can be a legitimate grief response. It is only when we associate feelings with losses that we begin to understand. How many of you, for instance, have watched someone (or maybe a pet) you loved die slowly and in a great deal of pain? Or cared for someone who through stroke or disease had lost their faculties long before dying? And when they died perhaps there was a little bit of relief, or even joy, that this loved one finally had been released from their suffering or incarceration. The feelings of sadness and upset are related to their dying and the fact that your life will never be the same. The feelings of relief and joy are related to losses such as not having to watch someone we love in continual pain anymore; no longer having difficulties which arose from not being able to communicate properly; no longer having the burden of visiting and caring and the subsequent changes to our own routine. When we acknowledge these, relief is an honest response.

But sometimes these are the emotions that we are not permitted to express in our society. When people do, they often discover just what an awful person they are for saying such things. Others hasten to assure them that 'They shouldn't feel like that' or to chastise them with a reminder of how selfish they are and to 'Think what (the deceased) would be feeling if they heard you saying these things'.

Comments of this nature impose guilt and shame which we are then left to wrestle with, and these feelings in particular have the effect of undermining what was a natural response. They complicate a normal grieving process. Such comments suggest that the speaker simply has not been through a similar process, or else hasn't found a way of expressing their own relief and consequently feels guilty when they see someone else doing so.

As we have discovered there are many losses associated with one big loss. Sometimes it takes a bit of figuring out which feelings belong to which losses. All are valid, for this is your experience alone. Having many emotions at the same time does not mean that you are abnormal, or going mad. It means that you are experiencing many different feelings all at the same time. Time, and a willingness on your part to sit and reflect on what is happening, will bring insight and growth beyond the point of 'stuckness' and the expectations of others. Alternatively it may be that some input from counselling could prove helpful. Far healthier for you to explore these feelings and give them expression than to squirrel them away.

Perceptions (or intellectual/mental responses):
- Disbelief (It didn't happen/There must be some mistake)
- Confusion • Preoccupation (With thoughts about the deceased or the lost 'object' [cause, situation, relationship]) • Heightened Awareness (A sense of presence of the deceased person) • Memory loss/Absent-mindedness • Inability to concentrate

How our intellectual processes are affected while we are grieving is also not fully recognised. Not many want to mention that they have forgotten the name of a most common object or can't remember a good friend's name. And heaven forbid if the boss found out about their diminished concentration span. Neither do most people feel comfortable talking about an 'after-death' experience they may have had with their deceased. As a consequence, we are unaware that what we experience are manifestations of grief and think instead that we may be losing our mind.

Having an after-death experience of the deceased is a most common occurrence, and is a quite normal and natural part of grief and grieving. It is to be expected following the death of someone close. Sadly, few people speak about this experience because our society is sometimes harsh in its response. More often than not such an experience is described as hallucinatory, and that in itself conjures up unpleasant connotations.

I prefer to refer to it as having an experience of the deceased. I had a wonderful experience of this when my mum died. It can happen in many different ways and when people have discovered that they can talk about it without fear of being judged, ridiculed or doubted, they usually express enormous relief and then fully accept and enjoy what has happened.

It may be that you felt the presence of the deceased. Others report hearing their voice, or seeing their loved one smile in a photograph suffused in soft light. I 'saw' my mum with her God and could tell that she was ecstatically happy. You may smell a particular scent, or you may sense a change in the temperature and just know that your loved one is right beside you. Some have told me about having vivid dreams where the deceased spoke to them and left a clear message. Others report waking suddenly to find the deceased watching over them.

If you have had such an experience I encourage you not to be dismissive of it. Share it with those whom you trust, and hang on to it. Don't let anyone belittle or take away what has happened for you. It is your experience.

This type of experience can happen quite spontaneously. It is different from, and I am not endorsing, seances. More often than not, the result leaves the survivor feeling reassured and more at peace, and with a very special memory. I've found when it has not been uplifting, there is usually more good-bye work to be done. The survivor or bereaved may still be angry with the deceased and need to work through that anger, or some other emotion or issue. A less than satisfying experience for the survivor is always indicative of unfinished business. If you have trouble identifying the nature of this unfinished business, this is the time to consider support through professional counselling.

Should someone share this type of experience with you, I suggest you avoid creating the kind of conversation that questions whether it could happen and how (which is what most people get into). Rather I encourage you to respond to that person's reality. What they have experienced, and the fact that they shared it with you, are both special and worthy of respect. Indeed it is sacred.

Others have a quite different experience. They may wake one day to realise they cannot remember what the deceased looked like, or they cannot recall specific detail about what it is they have now lost and which was special for them. This can happen quite suddenly, and as well as being frightening, it also induces feelings of guilt. It's unsettling not to be able to recall a loved one's voice or remember what a special place looked like.

Again, we know that it is normal for this to happen. You have done nothing to bring this about, and you are not going mad. There seems to be no apparent pattern to how long this memory loss will continue, but I have not worked with anyone yet who has not regained their capacity to remember.

Spirituality:

• Repeated Questioning (Why? Why me? Why now? Is there a God in the midst of this, and if so where?) • Seeking a greater meaning and purpose to what has happened • Re-defining values • Re-evaluating beliefs • Growing in self awareness

Whether we care to admit it or not, our spirituality is the very heart of us. And it is at the heart of our grief and grieving process. This is the part of us that always wants to ask 'why': why me, why now, why this way, why not them, why, why, why?

When the questions are spoken, the majority of people will respond in one of two ways. These responses are understandable, and are often motivated by good intentions, but usually aren't very effective. The first is to problem solve and try to offer a logical answer. The second is to offer platitudes in an attempt to make you feel better.

'Why' is not seeking a ready answer, nor is it wishing to be silenced. It is a passionate cry of anguish and is the start of a process that strives to gain some insight into how the world works and what life is all about. It seeks meaning and purpose and is a cry from the deepest most primal part of our being that needs connection with something which is infinite and greater than the grief that overwhelms us. Ask your 'why'. Speak it to the universe. How else are you to find the knowledge you seek?

I have learned much from my own experience concerning this. When I began working as a funeral director's assistant, the work was much as I expected. The majority of people I arranged funerals for and looked after in the mortuary were either elderly or had been very sick. I did not realise it then, but I had death firmly equated with sickness and old age. However, the day came when I was sent to collect the body of a baby from the morgue. I wept as I carried this precious bundle wrapped in cotton wool to the car and placed it on the front seat beside me. I found myself talking to this little one all the way back to work.

That was all I was required to do, but it was my first exposure to the harder reality of funeral directing. It was also all that I could manage at that time.

Later I raged; I remember going to the beach and walking for hours, screaming all my 'whys' to the waves and the wind and the seagulls. I don't remember expecting any answers but I felt a lot better after expressing what I perceived as the gross injustice of it all. Who had allowed this to happen, and did they really know what they were doing anyway? (I had a fine time at the beach. A lonely, isolated beach, I might add.)

Some days later I was surprised, and somewhat disconcerted to discover that my answer was within me. I have used it now to dedicate this book to my grand-nephews and niece. *You each are a note in the love song of creation; the harmony always is true.*

And slowly I began to understand that life is not a *given* and death will occur to us all. Some will live a long and sustained note, some will live the recognised measure, and yet others will live the time of the delicate, most fleeting of grace-notes that are essential to make any melody complete. And with this insight came the realisation that I no longer could take life for granted and that death is no respecter of our expectations. However, few of us begin to think about these things until we are faced with a death, or a crisis that has a real impact on our lives. Asking 'why' is how we confront what has happened and how we seek understanding. It is right and real that we should ask it.

Yet in doing so, many have feelings of guilt. Suddenly people find themselves questioning those very beliefs and values that have sustained them for a lifetime, or even a God who seems to have betrayed them. Still, ask your 'why', and continue to seek your answer. In the process of doing so you will discover a lot about yourself, and find courage you never knew you had. You may also, like I did, find knowing within you that will increase your spiritual awareness to a new and greater level of consciousness.

Behaviours:

• Disturbed sleeping pattern • Disturbed eating pattern • Altered sexual needs • Social withdrawal • Dreams of the deceased, or of what has been lost • Avoiding reminders of what has been lost, or the deceased • Searching and calling out • Sighing • Restless over-activity • Crying • Visiting places or carrying objects that are special reminders of the loss • Treasuring objects from the past • Angry outbursts

I have used the word disturbance in relation to sleeping and eating patterns. Disturbance means a change to what was previously a regular pattern – grief disturbs several patterns.

When grieving, some people eat more, some less. Some may be attracted to sweet foods or just find themselves drinking endless cups of tea or coffee. Some go right off their food and it becomes a real effort to eat. Food tastes like sawdust. Others find themselves eating little and often, rather than the regular three meals a day.

It is similar with sleeping patterns. Some people may sleep more than usual, others hardly at all. Some may sleep for an hour or two and not be able to sleep thereafter. Others find themselves dozing off in the middle of the day or falling into bed as soon as they have had tea.

More often than not, people find that their sexual needs also alter. They may want to have sex more, or less, or their sexual energy may become spasmodic or even non-existent. I have found the most common response is for people to want nurturing rather than sexual activity when grieving. Cuddles are wonderfully reassuring and provide security and comfort without demanding performance or energy that is not there to give. However any such change needs to be communicated to your partner. Explaining the change requires honesty and sensitivity. Be careful to avoid suggestions of blame or responsibility on their part. This will go a long way towards ensuring that your relationship continues in a loving, accepting and supportive way. It will also prevent possible misinterpretation with new liaisons while you are still vulnerable. All too frequently a lack of communication results in intimate contact when tenderness is all that is needed.

Although it can be frightening, anger is another normal reaction to loss and a natural part of the grieving process. Generally speaking, anger is not tolerated and few have learned how to express it in a healthy, constructive way. The tendency is to minimise anger by using less emotionally charged words, like 'irritation' or 'annoyance'. This tends to make anger more tolerable both to the individual and to their audience. Yet if the full extent of someone's anger is not faced, recovery is compromised.

Anger is an energy. It cannot be destroyed or forgotten. This angry energy has to be converted and given expression. It is helpful to recognise that anger is legitimate and does have some objectives:

- Anger registers a protest about what has happened. It is an attempt to ward off a reality which is seen as devastating, untimely and unwarranted.

- Anger is a means of retrieval, in that it continues to feed the hope that somehow what has happened can be reversed. Anger therefore craves a target, most usually the perceived author of the crisis.

- Anger is a form of control. It usually erupts when we feel helpless or powerless and is an emotional response that is designed to regain control. It is a defense against feeling impotent.

Underlying anger is the unconscious hope that somehow by conveying anger, all will be put right. It is only through giving it expression that a person comes to realise that no amount of anger will change the reality of what has happened.

However, given the conditioning that most of us have experienced, when anger legitimately surfaces as part of grief, few are able to give it direct expression, and anger is commonly perceived to be a personal shortcoming. Thus shame frequently accompanies anger. Consequently anger is denied.

Anger is also complex. Working through it can take time, and often what a person is angry with, or about, is not obvious. Anger needs to be broken down so that the person can come to define what they are angry about. It can be related to a subsequent or intrinsic loss that is not always immediately apparent, or the disappointment that results from expectations not being met. Skilled help may be needed to assist with this identification, and to learn effective, constructive methods for expressing the emotion. Anger must be confronted in order for the individual to achieve peace with what has happened.

Unexpressed anger leads to unresolved anger, which in turn leads to bitterness and sometimes depression. The only life it is then permitted is in substitute behaviours that admittedly are more socially acceptable, but which are costly, and destructive. Sarcasm, gossip, and criticism are all forms of an indirect expression of anger. They afford temporary relief by focusing on the shortcomings of someone else, and help people to avoid looking at their own problems. Unexpressed anger is also commonly displaced into psychosomatic based illnesses, and/ or depression. For some people it is more acceptable to go into a depressed state than to give expression to anger. But holding onto anger causes physical changes in the body that, when sustained, can produce many illnesses. It also causes a person to remain angry, because the anger is not being dealt with directly.

Anger is a natural response, so give yourself permission to acknowledge it. Share with those around you when you are angry (they will have read the signs anyway!), but avoid blaming or attacking them personally. Instead, direct your verbal attack to a cushion, or stuffed toy, or by writing about what is making you feel this way. Safe guidelines are – to not hurt yourself, nor anyone else, nor to destroy property.

As you can see, there is no right or wrong about these disturbances. They merely bring about a difference and that is okay. Do be aware of the changes however, and monitor what is happening for you. You may well find a new pattern developing and then be able to make some changes to accommodate this. It is usually when we ignore new differences and persist in trying to make previous demands fit around them, or vice versa, that difficulties arise. It is also important to keep an eye on how long these disturbances go on for. A lengthy period of not eating and disturbed sleep can have its own consequences and sometimes it is appropriate to make an intervention that will interrupt this tiring cycle. These disturbances can have physical consequences and a visit to your doctor or naturopath will provide assistance to cope with them. Like all the manifestations of grief, they will abate as we proceed with our grieving.

Summary

The most awful thing about grief is that it just arrives. The disturbances listed above just happen to you. And there is usually no rational explanation to help you understand what you are experiencing, and you'll also discover that you are unable to control it. Intense feelings will often wash over you like waves, and in the most public of places or at the most inappropriate times, and you can do nothing about it. It is embarrassing and frustrating and you feel powerless. Despite giving yourself positive messages and believing you should be over it by now, you continue to experience ups and downs in your moods, tiredness that is often extreme, and are forever thinking about the someone or something you have lost. All too frequently these symptoms and the accompanying sadness are confused with depression.

Because all of this is so frightening, and we are neither able to explain nor control it, people often think there is something wrong with them, and that they going mad. But you (and they) are not mad. Neither are you bad or stupid. You have survived a traumatic event that has resulted in loss and which is cause for you to experience grief.

What you are experiencing is normal.

But its a lot more than just sadness.

Food For Thought

Falling Apart

I seem to be falling apart
My attention span can be measured in seconds
My patience in minutes
I cry at the drop of a hat
I forget things constantly
The morning toast burns daily
I forget to sign the cheques
Half of everything in the house is misplaced
Feelings of anxiety and restlessness are my constant
    companions
Rainy days seem extra dreary
Sunny days seem an outrage
Other people's pain and frustration seem insignificant
Laughing, happy people seem out of place in my world
It has become routine to feel half crazy
I am normal I am told
I am a newly grieving person.

Eloise Cole

Personal Reflection

Take time now to consider your own reality. List everything you have noticed lately, and those things you are only now becoming aware of. Take your time, and keep adding until it is just right for you. Honour not only what you have written, but also the experience it comes from. Respect also the courage you have that is enabling you to complete this work.

Physical Sensations:

Perceptions:

Feelings:

Spiritual Awareness:

Behaviours:

Summary of Key Points

- We experience grief physically, intellectually, emotionally and spiritually.

- Asking 'why' is the way we begin to confront our new reality and seek a new perspective that helps us to understand what is happening to us. It is important to ask why.

- Grief and sadness are often confused with depression.

- Relief is a legitimate grief response.

- Having many feelings at the same time does not mean that you are going mad. It means that you are having several different feelings at the same time.

- It is important to communicate what you are experiencing and your changing needs to your partner.

- If behavioural changes persist for a lengthy time, or become physically taxing, it is appropriate to seek assistance from your doctor or naturopath.

- You are not mad or bad if you are feeling awful. Neither are you being stupid. You are probably experiencing disenfranchised grief, which means that either your loss or your grief has not been recognised.

- It is not selfish to grieve.

4 *Myth: Everyone should grieve the same way*

> *Reality: Our grieving is as unique as we are.*

No two people will grieve in the same way. Even when two people experience the same loss, in similar circumstances, they will react differently. Certainly the general features will be familiar to many who have had a major loss in their lives. But your grief, and more particularly, the way you express that grief, will be as unique as you are. Even within a family, siblings can experience a common loss, say in the death of their parent, and each will be affected and respond differently.

So what accounts for this? Why is it that for one person grief and grieving may last a very short time, while another seems to struggle forever? Why is it that for some, grief is a very intense experience, and yet for others it seems to be only a fleeting inconvenience? What is it that enables some people to grieve when the loss occurs, while others wait, sometimes for years, to begin the process? Part of the answer lies in our attitude. But how do we develop our attitudes toward loss and grief and how do we address and change them if they don't work for us?

Grieving, although a natural process, is a complex phenomena. Rather than endeavour to understand it, or develop appropriate means through which to deal with it, our society by and large has tended to minimise and stereotype grief with the myths I hope to dispel. To dispel the myth of this chapter we need to explore the determinants of grief.

There are many factors that determine how an individual will grieve, but they can be grouped into three main areas:

- The circumstances (including personality and personal history) surrounding the loss or death
- How grief is dealt with in our family system
- Our personal growth and development

The circumstances surrounding the loss or death

This group of determinants relates to the who, what, when, where, and how of things and can be placed in context as follows:

- Who has died, or what was the loss
- The nature of the attachment
- How the loss occurred
- Our personal history of loss
- Individual personality differences
- Social support

1. Who has Died, or What Was the Loss

First of all, we grieve quite differently for the loss of a parent than we do for the loss of a child. Again, we grieve differently for the loss of a sibling than we do for a partner or spouse. Similarly, someone will grieve in a different way for the loss of a body part than they will for the loss of a house, job, family pet or object. And secondly, the degree of reaction is brought about by the amount of emotional investment we have had in whoever or whatever has been lost. And the combination of these two factors will be very different for everybody.

As already discussed, it is never helpful to make assumptions about the nature of any loss that someone else has experienced. Only the person who is experiencing the loss can determine its significance for them. I remember one young man of around 19 years who I counselled, and whose case illustrated this point well. He was deeply distressed at the recent death of his grandmother, not quite six months previously. He was also hurt and confused by the responses he was encountering both from his friends and in his workplace. He was being criticised quite openly for his transparent grief, because it was 'only' his grandmother who had died, and it had been six months ago. As well as the hurt and confusion, he was also feeling like an outcast who was not understood. And, of course, he was feeling guilty as a result of these accusations. He did not know what to do but knew that he wanted desperately to honour his grandmother and grieve her leaving him.

In a very short space of time I learned how important this relationship was to him. I also discovered that his parents had separated when he was just two years old, and that he had lived with his grandparents ever since. Suddenly one begins to realise that his grandmother was not only grandmother but surrogate mother as well. In effect, it was as if he had two losses. The grief he experienced was in accordance with these losses. He needed to grieve as one would for the death of a mum, and all that relationship had encompassed. And he also needed to grieve for the death of his grandmother. And so we did just that; without the negative messages that suggested any short-coming on his part.

In other circumstances we may have to work equally hard to understand a person's reaction, or lack of it. It may be that another 19-year-old tells you, with about as much interest as if he were discussing the weather, that his grandmother has just died. Rather than racing to condemn him for his lack of sympathy or respect, I would suggest asking a few questions that will reveal the nature of the relationship. It may be that he has never met his grandmother. Perhaps his parents immigrated to this country before he was born and he has never known any of his extended family. In this case his grandmother may simply be a face in a photo album. And there is only a limited amount of emotional involvement you can invest in that. His response then would be perfectly appropriate.

We may not understand why someone is grieving but we can ask if they want to talk about it. We can also ask why the loss is so important, or what it means to that person. And then we listen. With all of our being, we listen to what that person is telling us. We do not then put our point of view, or offer our opinion, or share a similar experience. We do not have to be critical or make a judgement about what they are saying or of how they may be grieving. We just listen, and in so doing we will come to appreciate who, or what, they have lost and just what it means to them. And thus we will gain some insight into their grieving behaviour.

2. The Nature of the Attachment

Once we know who the person was (or what has been lost) and what meaning that has, we can begin to understand something about the nature of the attachment. This includes knowing about:

- The strength of the attachment
- What it provided and
- What degree of ambivalence was involved

The strength of the attachment can range anywhere along a continuum from intense to very weak. Any number of factors will have influenced the strength of this attachment and it is rarely helpful to make assumptions about them. We just need to be able to accept that the severity of one's grief increases in proportion to the intensity of the love relationship.

A sense of security is most commonly provided by attachment. Therefore, knowing what a particular relationship provided in the way of security is also important in order to understand how someone might grieve. Take work for example. For some their identity is connected to the work they do, so that when faced with redundancy, it is a lot more than just a job they are losing. The loss of self-esteem, confidence, and a sense of belonging, meaning and purpose will all be casualties. More often than not they will perceive themselves as being a failure because they now have no professional role with which to identify themselves.

Similarly, if a survivor has needed the deceased, or now absent partner, to provide them with a sense of self-esteem or well-being, (in other words to make them feel complete) then the separation will be acute and the grief intense and prolonged.

Ambivalence is a natural part of any close relationship and means that we can (and do) have opposing or quite contradictory feelings at times. This is commonly experienced as the old love/hate relationship. Usually the positive feelings far outweigh any negative ones but in the case of a highly ambivalent relationship – where the negative feelings co-exist in equal proportions or exceed the positive ones – there is always a more difficult grief reaction.

I was approached during a workshop once by a woman who I estimated to be in her fifties. She told me that both her parents had died when she was a child and that she had struggled ever since with her feelings toward them. The feelings she had for each parent were very different and she considered these feelings to be not only abnormal, but wrong, and certainly not the way any person should feel after their parents had died. She had carried a great deal of guilt about this for a long time. As a result she was convinced that she was not a very nice person and that she would be punished for her awful feelings when she died. We agreed to work together for a period of time.

She began by talking about the relationship she had with her mum. There was plenty in what she said that suggested that it had been healthy, positive, and loving. She also mentioned very quietly, and with her eyes downcast, that she had a lot of anger toward her mum. I did not question the reason for this just then. It was enough that she was aware of it, and to me this ambivalence was realistic in a healthy relationship.

The feelings she expressed toward her dad were quite different and were revealed more slowly. She was aware of being angry, bitter, resentful, full of hatred, and pleased that he was dead, and as much as she tried to find some, there was no love. Immediately I began to wonder at the relationship she had with her father and what exactly she had lost when he died. Very gently I began to explain this to her – that our feelings reflect our losses – and then I asked her what she had lost when her dad died.

Quiet reflection of the question resulted in her sobbing. She had, she struggled to tell me, lost a man who was drunk more often than not; who had ruled the house with violence and fear; and who had abused her sexually for most of her childhood. And suddenly amidst the tears she smiled at me and explained that she could see that her feelings had a legitimate source. Until this point she had always supposed that because he was her father she should feel sorry for his dying. Now she had a different framework with which to understand what was happening. She was then able to identify very quickly the source of her anger toward her mum as 'Where were you when I needed you?'

The relationships this woman had with her mother and father were very different. She was strongly attached to each, but for different reasons. Each provided something different in terms of security, identity and love. And each reflected an ambivalence that had induced guilt and which had kept her stuck in her grief for many years.

3. How the Loss Occurred

How a person has died, or how the loss occurred, also has something to do with how we will grieve. Disasters, death or loss that have been sudden, unexpected or traumatic, result in grief that can be profound and long-term, and a complicated recovery process for survivors. This is because so many other factors come into play.

Disaster, or traumatic loss is invariably untimely. It can result in multiple deaths that are often violent, damaging or mutilating, and this aspect adds further stress to the survivor. The event may be surrounded in uncertainty, bodies may not be recovered, or there may be difficulties with identification, viewing and other good-bye work that can not be completed.

Frequently this kind of event attracts press attention and although this may mobilise public sympathy and support, more often than not it also means that the private aspects of loss cannot be kept private. This can lead to the bereaved/survivors putting a protective banner around themselves. Public attention and care may be well-intentioned, yet may be rejected because it is overwhelming or because normal skills that enable response are dulled. Personal losses may be extremely difficult to acknowledge if others seem to have lost more. Despite the fact that one person's loss may be overwhelming, that will be difficult to admit if press and public seem to be comparing losses and suggesting that 'There are other people worse off than you'.

It also means that there are public expectations about response and behaviour that don't necessarily fit with the bereaved, or survivors' needs. The expression of grief may be temporarily set aside as survival issues are often critical in these circumstances. These losses that are sudden, traumatic or the result of disasters are frequently perceived as being unfair or unjust. And because guilt and anger are often prominent there is the desperate search for 'someone to blame'.

A death or loss that carries a social stigma also makes for an intense and often complicated grieving process. Having a stigma attached to the loss suggests there is some disgrace or reproach involved, and the survivor often feels shame because of this social response. Death by suicide, abortion or AIDS unfortunately still carry a degree of stigma. This can mean those left to grieve have a lonely time of it and often lack the social support they need.

A further circumstantial aspect of loss that influences grieving is where the loss occurred. Our physical proximity has a bearing on whether it is possible to view the place of the accident or death, or to attend funeral services, or even to return the body of the loved one to the survivors. When distance prevents any one of these factors being attended to, there is little to assist the grieving process or facilitate recovery.

4. Our Personal History of Loss

Previous experience always affects the way we cope with our present losses. When a person's major loss has been shelved or not adequately resolved, for whatever reason, the unfinished business of that loss becomes part of the current grief response. Sometimes this can be overwhelming, especially if there have been many losses stored away. We can actually become stuck in our grief simply because of overload.

I remember working with a woman who had reached just such a point. She came to see me because she was aware she had lost touch with her feelings, but didn't understand why.

We made a profile of her losses for the previous ten years. We listed only the obvious, major losses. The list included the following: dissolution of marriage, loss of children as they elected to stay with their father, change of country, death of sister, death of sister's son (her nephew) by suicide, death of parents, death of a grandparent, changes of jobs, houses and communities, death of a much loved pet, death of another sibling. When she saw the list she began to appreciate just what she had been through, and to realise that her bodily system had sought to safeguard itself from so much pain and induced a numbness. It wasn't until we looked back over her life and did this review that she was able to appreciate what was happening for her and that she was emotionally exhausted.

This example may appear extreme but many people suffer multiple losses in their lives. Seldom do losses wait until we are prepared. It pays to check what has happened previously for the person concerned, or to look into their present circumstances in order to appreciate what it is they might be coping with.

5. Individual Personality Differences

Quite simply, we are all different. We know that we are all born with a physical genetic code that is unique. Who we are, and how we express ourselves emotionally and psychologically, are equally unique. This in itself accounts for why one person sees joy where another sees sorrow. Our life experiences also mould us, as do our culture, attitudes, beliefs, and what we have been taught. It is helpful to reflect on what has happened in our history that might influence the way we currently respond.

We will all have developed different strategies of coping. Mostly we deal with grief by using the same coping mechanism we use to manage other difficulties in our lives. Some of these are identified in 'Food For Thought' on page 89. However there is an endless number of ways that we come to cope with life, and this also accounts for the differences we perceive in how people grieve. We can blame others for our loss, or appear helpless and assume the role of victim. We can develop a martyr complex, or avoid people. We can strive to be perfect in everything we do until the fear of not being perfect paralyses. We can simply refuse to talk. The list is endless. And I am not implying criticism in identifying some of them.

The challenge is to identify what strategies we may have developed earlier in life that assisted us in some way, but which have now outlived their usefulness and are preventing us from grieving. The way to start this process is to identify not only what strategy we employ, but in what circumstances we use it, and why we find it necessary. The goal is to foster a new strategy for coping that is more appropriate behaviour for us as adults and which will help our grieving process.

Life involves a series of losses or changes and it stands to reason that we will all be grieving to a smaller or larger degree throughout our lives. The way we respond will be personal. When we move beyond the expectation that everyone should respond in the same way, it brings an awareness that tolerates individual differences.

6. Social Support

There are times when you will need to be alone, and to keep your grief private. Paradoxically however, grieving is a social process. Your grieving can never be fully resolved without the input of others. We need people to listen to us, care for us, challenge us, inspire us, support us, comfort us, teach us new skills, exchange ideas with and to share this most painful part of our journey with them. How else are we to know that we can survive? Unfortunately the most commonly held view is supported by yet another myth that suggests 'You should be able to do this on your own'.

It is well established that those people who have healthy social networks progress through their grieving more rapidly than those who do not. Good friends assist, almost unwittingly, simply by being present throughout and allowing grief to be expressed. For many however, especially the elderly, there is not constant support. And for others, like the intellectually disabled, there is frequently a lack of understanding of knowing how to help them in their grieving. And yet others are denied either recognition, support or understanding as society offers judgement rather than compassion.

Yet the final phase of grieving is about enjoying life again. And we definitely need people to help us to do that. Those people who refuse to involve another, or who do not have someone else they can involve, struggle to express their grief and are more inclined to adapt by learning to live with it, rather than moving on from it. And so our social connections, or lack of them, is another vital aspect that influences grieving.

Family Systems

Primarily we learn to cope with grief by what is modelled in our family. We may never have been consciously taught about grief or what to do about it, but we will have learnt well enough from what has happened around us. There will have been a particular way that family crises were dealt with, and we will have become familiar with that pattern of behaviour. Unfortunately, I have discovered that only rarely do people ever question the appropriateness of the family behaviour and their subsequent learning. Rather they believe instead that what they have been exposed to is the only way of approaching grief, and they continue to adhere to behavioural patterns even when they prove to be unhelpful.

As a child you may have been sent to stay with neighbours when a family death occurred because someone sought to protect you. What many unconsciously learn when this happens, is to distance themselves from death and all that accompanies it. All too frequently children are taught to cope with death by replacement. When nothing is discussed, and no explanations given, a child learns not to talk about things or to show their feelings. And these are the tools with which they now attempt to deal with loss and grief, death and bereavement, as adults.

My experiences have shown me that families adopt common patterns in order to cope with grief. Research has also identified that the same patterns are widely used. These patterns are modelled from generation to generation, which ensures their perpetuation. You may recognise one or more of the following strategies as ones used in your family.

- Let's not talk about it. Death is a taboo subject and silence is the only way to cope. This style is usually adopted when the parents themselves have unresolved grief from the death of their parents, or children. Major losses and the grief it precipitates are never discussed.

- Someone must be responsible for this. One or more persons are sought out to blame for what has happened. It has the effect of making others feel guilty and is usually the result of the parents wanting revenge or to rigidly control everything. Loss and grief are always someone else's fault and the aggrieved become victims.

- The Stiff-Upper-Lip-Brigade. Any feelings or distress are carefully concealed and intimate relationships are avoided. There is a belief that letting people get close to you is risky and will be dangerous. Losses are not acknowledged and grief is suppressed, as is compassion.

- Pretend nothing has happened. Life must continue as before and there is no flexibility. The gap that is left by the loss, or death, is filled immediately to maintain the status quo. Grief is avoided so the system won't be undermined and nothing (and nobody) will have to change.

- This is the end. There is chaos when loss occurs and often the family fragments. There are no strong links within the family and usually other support networks are limited or non-existent. Individuals have few personal resources with which to cope and many have had other major losses in their lives, such as divorce, or mental illness. Loss and grief are considered a catastrophe and dramatised, and are frequently the straws that break the camel's back.

- We must do this right. Doing 'it' right is more important than attending to anything else. Individual needs and feelings are not important. Fear is the driving force. Intellectualising everything and everyone is the main way of coping. Loss and grief take a back seat to 'impression management'.

- We can share anything and we are okay. In this family there is open and honest sharing of feelings. Positive and negative feelings are tolerated, as is the fact that each member is responding differently to what has happened. Members are intimate with one another and share their distress. Losses are respected and grieving is resolved through mutual care and consolation.

There is nothing that can protect us from loss or the pain it brings. It is part of life. Like every other aspect of life, we need to learn how to respond and develop personal responsibility in the face of it. It is only the last of the strategies listed above that will assist us to accept and then resolve our grief. The others offer ways to avoid, deny, and control it. They may offer some relief in the short term, but they do not help to resolve the grief, and the long-term task for anyone who uses these methods is to learn to live with their grief. And many do, because loyalty to early learning and family members holds strong. These myths have been invented to support this misplaced loyalty!

Personal Growth and Development

We seldom pause to consider what is meant by personal growth, and all too frequently development is a term that is synonymous with workplace training programmes. Personal growth is just that: our individual growth as a person. Because they look like adults, and dress and talk like adults, many grown-ups think there is little left in the way of growth to do. After all, they are old enough, hold responsible jobs and have professional qualifications. However, according to Abraham Maslow* only two percent of grown-ups are 'self-actualised' – that is, free to be themselves and be what they want.

Being an adult involves having ideals and principles, and the character to stick to them, and yet being flexible enough to review and change as you evolve. It means having a system of personal values and being clear about why you hold to them. It means that your self-esteem is internally sourced and not dependent on the approval of others. It means that you are able to trust yourself and your intuition and embrace your emotions without resistance. Being adult means you take personal responsibility for yourself and creating your own life rather than manipulating or hurting others to get your own way. Adults live happy and fulfilled lives and are able to engage fully in love that supports the spiritual growth of another. Self-actualisation is personal responsibility based on self awareness,

---

* Abraham Maslow (1908–1970) is generally accepted as the father of humanistic/existential therapy. His theories have had a strong impact on pastoral and educational counselling. He believed that the process of personality development is akin to growth.

self-esteem and self-acceptance. Self-actualisation correlates to our level of spirituality.

So how does this come about? A lot of people never achieve this stage of development. There are four parts to our being: the physical, intellectual, emotional and spiritual. And we need to grow in each of these aspects of our being. Usually they are depicted like this:

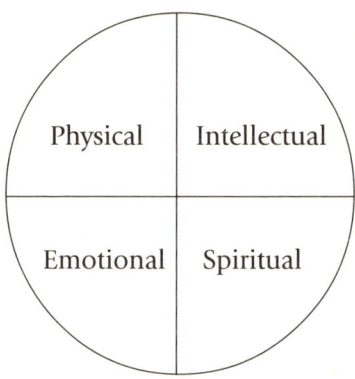

This gives the impression that these four aspects of our being are divided up neatly and equally into the established quota, or quarter. I believe it is more complex. In each of these quadrants we grow at different rates, at different times in our lives, and for different reasons.

Growth in our physical sphere occurs from birth and happens quite naturally. It is affected, of course, by the way we nurture the body, if we exercise it, and by our genes. We seldom pause to consciously think about what we have to do in order to grow physically. Around the age of 21 we discover that we are full grown. We have reached our possible maximum (that is, unless we have some illness or disability that prevents us from doing so). From this point we may grow outwards, but not upwards. But if we are to continue to function at maximum potential, we do need to become conscious about attending to our physical well-being.

Intellectual growth is somewhat different, and involves more than just academic achievement. But how much and what we know will be related to how open we have been to learning and expanding our mind. It includes having developed the ability to analyse and reason and problem solve. It also requires us to explore our own beliefs critically and move beyond our conditioning. It means we are able to be self-directed in our learning, change our style of learning to suit various situations and stay open to pursuing any opportunity that will extend our thinking and life philosophy. Life experiences can contribute to growth in this area. But note that there is a very big difference between having sixty years of life experience and living one year of life experience sixty times.

We have grown emotionally when we know what we are feeling at any time, know what that feeling is telling us, know what to do in response and are able to share our feelings with another. That is a lot of knowing, and a very complex process. Most people also realise that in revealing their feelings they make themselves vulnerable and uncomfortable, so it is the one thing they avoid doing, and thus never learn how to give appropriate expression to their feelings. The family system that we have grown up in will also have influenced our emotional growth. It is the likes of meditation, self-reflection and counselling that fosters growth. But unless and until we develop the capacity to have feelings and express ourselves, we remain emotionally stunted.

Spiritual growth is different from religious affiliation. Spirituality is the very core of us that begins to wonder and question what life is all about, why we are here, is there a universal power or life after death, and why, why, why. It is that part of us where we relate to ourselves, to others, and to the universe. It is about coming to know who you are and loving that. Religion can provide formalised answers to these types of questions, each slightly different in their appeal. But however we go about it, growth in this quadrant is marked by moving beyond any need to control, avoid, or deny anything. It is ironic, but natural enough, that most of us begin to ask these questions and only start our spiritual quest when we are faced with a crisis. Loss, death and grief are all forms of such a crisis.

Although brief and perhaps simplistic, the above explanation serves our purpose well enough. We have now defined being adult and how to achieve this state. If we look at ourselves closely, there will be noticeable differences in our growth in each dimension at, say, 21 years of age, and our growth at the moment. There is no right or wrong about this; it merely reflects how we changed in response to our experience and opportunities. The extent of our growth at any given time equates directly to the resources we call on when we engage with life. We can define growth as a measure of the ability we possess to cope with, or respond to, life events: In other words, this is our 'response ability', or our ability to be responsible.

For example, here is how I see my development at age 21.

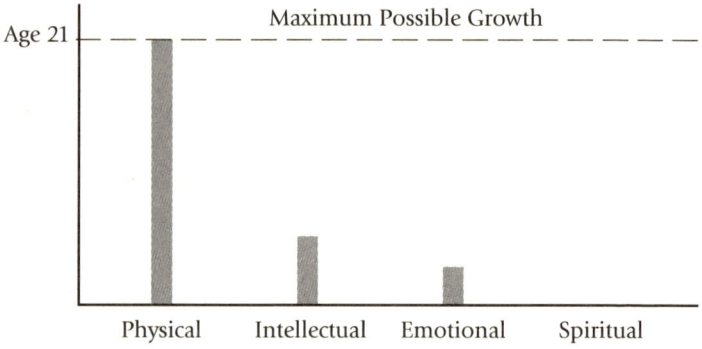

- Physically, I had reached my potential; I had grown all I was going to grow.

- Intellectually, I considered myself to be a failure and stupid: I had failed school certificate.

- Emotionally, I did not know what I felt or how to express feelings; I had learned to survive by suppressing them.

- Spiritually, I had avoided many opportunities to reflect on life issues. I lived my life to please others, and had not begun to shape my own identity.

When I plot this graph now, thirty plus years on, it looks different, and I think, a tad healthier.

- A diminishment of physical health represents the onset of arthritis and a need for hip replacements.

- The last 20 years have seen me gain several academic achievements and learn how to apply the knowledge – wisdom in my old age. Intellectually I feel more secure.

- Therapy, professional training and the completion of my own grief work means I am now friends with my feelings.

- And I am now my own person with a philosophy that affords me principles to live my life and with which to face death. I have experienced growth in the spiritual quadrant.

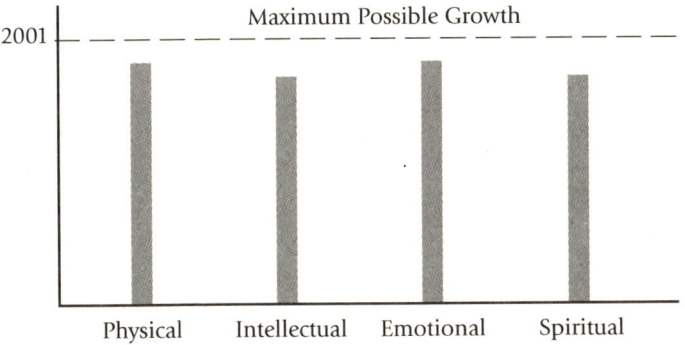

Still not perfect, with room to grow. But now when I face any life event, I have far more resources with which to respond. My growth is more balanced, and I can choose which response I will make. This is maturity, and what it means to be adult.

One key thing we need to understand, is that the development of our personal resources determines our ability to grieve. People will seek to cope with their grief by functioning out of whichever aspect of their personality is most well-developed. After all, that behaviour is what they are most familiar with and they know how to carry it out well. It also means that in those quadrants where there is little growth they will have limited resources with which to attend to their grieving. So here is further insight into why we each grieve differently. And why in some cases, grieving is never completed.

Grief is always experienced physically. Irrespective of our growth in other areas, we always carry the effects of grief in our bodies. As illustrated throughout, this is not well recognised and therefore physical manifestations of grief are dealt with medically, more often than not. Conversely, when growth in other areas is restricted, physicality will be the prominent means through which grief is expressed. Some will use strenuous physical exercise to attempt to alleviate their discomfort, while for others it is channelled into physical aggression.

When intellectual growth is dominant, people will intellectualise their grief. They will analyse it, moralise it, justify it, rationalise it and legalise it. They will go over and over everything in their minds. If, but, when, how and maybe, get worked to death (excuse the pun). Very little is ever resolved because grief can not be controlled like this. But the person is doing what they know best, and using their intellect will have been a powerful attribute that provided resolutions in the past. Unfortunately it seldom allows them to move forward and engage in the grieving process.

For someone who is well-developed emotionally, their response is somewhat different. They will be in touch with their feelings and express them quite naturally. When they are sad they will cry and experience no shame or embarrassment about doing so. If they are angry they will say so and find a constructive way to express it, and then move on. They may not be interested in the whys and wherefores about what has happened. But their feelings will guide them intuitively to do what they need to do in order to complete their grieving.

People who have grown strong in their spirituality will have a life philosophy or map from which they operate and which usually gives them great faith and courage, particularly in times of crisis. It's not that they don't question anything, because as we have discovered, they do. But they seem to have some deeper meaning or understanding which helps them to accept things. They are upset and yet somehow at peace with themselves. They are able to accept how life unfolds and refrain from personalising any crisis.

And so when any group of people share a common loss it becomes complex. Each member has difficulty in understanding why everyone is not reacting the same way they are. In fact each person will experience the loss differently because each has grown in a different way. One may intellectualise things, while another is very much in touch with their feelings. What makes it difficult is that neither can comprehend why the other is not responding in the same manner that they are. The thinker accuses the other of being over emotional and too demonstrative; the emotionally developed accuses the thinker of being callous, or unfeeling. And so on. When someone has developed spiritually, their response is different again. And if someone has not attended to the issues that promote their own growth in this area, they will tend to be dismissive of the responses of someone else who has. There is little communication among the group members, for each is speaking a different language and is unable to recognise and explain this to the other. The result all too often is disruptive while each blames the other for being unsympathetic to their needs.

I hope this sheds a little enlightenment. When there is a conflict of responses in a group of people, it doesn't mean that anyone is deliberately being difficult or unreasonable or insensitive. They are just doing what they can with the know-how they have got. It just happens to be different.

Summary

There are many factors that influence how a person will grieve. There are circumstances surrounding the loss that will have their own impact. How we have witnessed grief being dealt with in the past will also influence our responses as we automatically revert to learned behaviour. How aware we are of our personal growth and make-up also influences how we cope.

Grief affects us physically, intellectually, emotionally and spiritually. And we need to grow in each of these quadrants of our being in order to grieve and resolve our grief. Conversely, attending to our grieving demands input from us physically, intellectually, emotionally and spiritually. For this reason, grieving helps us grow to health and wholeness.

The combination of these factors can be experienced in a myriad of ways, and is why no two people grieve in quite the same form. To have an expectation that 'we should all grieve the same way' is at the least naïve. To insist that someone should grieve the same way you are is punitive.

Everyone is unique. And so is their grieving.

Food For Thought

People can truly believe that everyone is unique, and therefore has the need to grieve in their own way and at their own time. But their behaviour often belies this. Consider the following beliefs that people articulate. And then reflect on the behaviour they engage in.

Beliefs	Behaviour
People need to talk about their grief.	Avoid mentioning the loss or death.
Grieving has no time limit.	Express surprise when someone talks about their loss 6–12–18 months later.
Individual cultural and religious beliefs need to be respected.	Express their own beliefs strongly in disagreement with another.
It is acceptable to talk about the deceased.	Avoid referring to the deceased by name.
It is natural to cry.	Avoid saying anything that might upset the other.
I am sincere and genuine in responding to grieving people.	Use clichés when responding: e.g. you'll get over it, more fish in the sea.

Beliefs *cont'd*

Anger is part of grief
and needs to be vented
constructively.

It is important to work
through grief at your
own pace.

There will be a period of
adjustment during which
the person will need to
find new solutions to be
independent.

Grieving people need
to repeat their story and
be listened to.

Feelings need to be
acknowledged.

Behaviour *cont'd*

Feel uncomfortable or
embarrassed and find an
excuse to end the conver-
sation or leave when anger
emerges.

Arrange for a person to
socialise when they have
expressed a preference not to.

Take on responsibility
for some aspect of their
adjustment and then feel
trapped because they are
relied upon.

Tell their own experience,
or someone else's that is
similar.

Tell person they shouldn't
feel guilty (or that way) and
use logical argument to
explain why.

Personal Growth and Development Chart

Consider carefully and honestly your growth, or state of health, in each quadrant. Refer to the criteria described in this chapter and how it relates to being adult. While maximum possible growth has not been defined, be conscious of the effort you have made, opportunities taken, and the mindfulness with which you have nurtured your own growth. What is your 'response ability'? (See page 71 for an explanation of this term) Is it responsible, and all that you would like it to be? Do you feel that you have choices and are in control of your life? Or is your behaviour to any situation robot-like with little awareness?

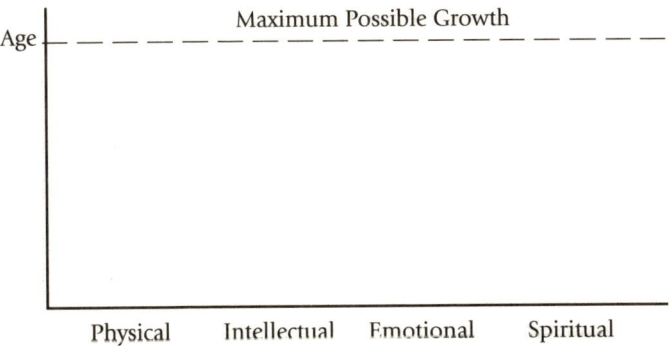

What is one area that you wish to develop?

What is the first step you will take to do this?

Summary of Key Points

- No two people will grieve in the same way.

- How a person will grieve is determined by
    - the circumstances surrounding the loss,
    - how they have witnessed their family deal with grief,
    - and their personal growth or 'response ability'.

- Individual differences in grieving need to be tolerated, not criticised.

- Grief is a private thing. Grieving is a social process.

- Often the strategies we learned as children or adolescents for managing loss and grief are inadequate or inappropriate for us as adults.

- We are responsible for nurturing our physical, intellectual, emotional and spiritual growth.

- People grow at different rates, at different times, for different reasons in each quadrant of their being.

- People seek initially to control their grief by functioning from that quadrant which is most well-developed.

- Grieving encourages our physical, intellectual, emotional and spiritual growth and well-being.

5 Myth: *Time will heal.*

Reality: *Time alone does not heal grief.*

Now is the time when we come to appreciate that there is a very big difference between grief and grieving. Grief is everything that we have discussed so far. It is all those manifestations earlier described which just arrive and affect us physically, mentally, emotionally and spiritually. This grief is our initial and natural response to a loss. It is involuntary. Grieving, on the other hand, is what we do in order to resolve this grief. Notice that it is a verb, a doing word, and therefore requires some input on our part. Grieving is not a passive process where we just wait until we feel better. Although this is in fact what most people do. This myth has held sway for so long and is so entrenched in our society that it has become a way of life.

The Snowstorm

I like to illustrate the difference between grief and grieving with something everyone can relate to. I use the model of a snowstorm. Picture those ornaments that are made of glass, somewhat like a bubble, which have a scene inside them – and when it is picked up and shaken a snowstorm is created. When someone experiences a major loss it is as if they have been picked up and shaken so that everything inside them has been churned about in a similar way. It is as if they are at the centre of the snowstorm. Everything they have known, everything that was familiar, has been disrupted and obliterated. White-out conditions. Life during this initial phase of grief is concentrated on surviving. Day by day. Sometimes moment by moment.

Consider what is happening when someone is experiencing this snowstorm. Regular sleeping patterns have changed; don't feel like eating properly; aching all over; tired all the time; can't concentrate, even to read a magazine; apt to fly off the handle at the smallest upset; constantly making silly mistakes with the simplest of tasks; wanting people to offer comfort and yet when they are around wanting them to be gone. We feel affronted that the world seems to continue as normal without noticing either us, or the crisis that has befallen us. The thought of getting up every morning to face another day is so horrendous that thoughts of suicide may preoccupy us. And the effort it requires to actually get up is so enormous that we have no energy left to do anything for the rest of the day, except try to survive. Never underestimate how devastating and debilitating an experience it can be for people in this snowstorm, or the effect it may have on them.

The snowstorm takes some time to settle, and so does the

initial disorientation. Given time however, the number of mani-festations and their intensity decreases. Bad weather does not last forever, and the snowstorm begins, quite naturally, to abate. Just when, varies enormously between individuals, but it is at this stage that people begin to feel slightly better. This settling of the snowstorm, gives the illusion of the grief having gone away, or that they 'must be getting over it'. 'Time is healing', they think.

However, it does not mean that life gets back to normal. It does mean that those overwhelmingly intense feelings are beginning to lose their edge and that our behaviour patterns may begin to adjust back to what we have been used to. Each day, although often still meaningless, is a little less frighten-ing. You may suddenly realise that a whole morning has passed without your having thought about what has happened. You might go a whole day without crying. You may even have found something to laugh about. If this is the case, there is no need to feel guilty or disloyal about having done so. You are begin-ning to experience that life does indeed continue after death or major loss.

But not in the same way. Life can never be the same as it was. And this is the time when the hard work of grieving begins. Just how we do this is the subject of the next chapter. It is im-portant that we now move on to do this hard work, for two key reasons. First, because only the work of grieving will do away with the snowstorm. When this is not done it's as if we continue to carry our snowstorm with us – and it can be easily shaken again by any incident or remark that reminds us of our loss.

Keeping busy, avoiding things or people that remind us of what has happened, not talking or trying not to think about how we are really feeling – all of these things create the illusion that we are getting better, and they also keep any future snow-storm at bay. People can live like this for long periods of time and actually learn to live with the pain that is in their hearts and to ignore the pain that is in their bodies, or tolerate it as normal. They can become expert at avoiding people's questions about their health or the loss they have experienced, and divert general conversation when it becomes uncomfortable. They may find a myriad of ways to suppress their feelings and not let them show. But none of these strategies will help them (or us) to actually deal with grief and prevent further snowstorms. Rather they are all subtle forms of denial and avoidance.

We need to grieve. Life can become frightening, restricted and have a very narrow focus when we avoid everything that may cause pain or memories to flood into our consciousness. We need to do our grieving in order to integrate this experience and get on with the business of enjoying life and living again.

How we go about integrating these major life experiences is covered more fully in subsequent chapters. It is sufficient to acknowledge here that grieving helps us to adjust and move forward in our lives. We learn and grow because of it. When the loss involves other people, either by separation or death, it becomes even more important that we do the hard work of grieving because it is the very means by which we disentangle from relationships. Unless and until we disengage from the relationship as we have known it, neither party is free to move on and create a new experience. Instead people tend to live with regrets and bitterness, and hang onto the 'if onlys' and 'what ifs'. When death is involved, the bereft are not free to move forward and enjoy their current phase of life. The 'old' needs to be concluded, and a 'new' established. This is change, and the very process of life. But not to adapt, or to seek to preserve the past when change has occurred, is to stagnate. And it affects more than just you. This second reason for the need to grieve is not so well-known and somewhat more controversial, and as mentioned, this theme will be developed more fully.

As an illustration I offer the following snapshot. An elderly woman once approached me at the end of a lecture I had given. She explained that her baby had been stillborn 58 years ago. She also explained that people had told her time would heal. 'Well, excuse me please' she said, 'but I have been waiting 58 years for the pain to go away and be healed. And it never has. I am still waiting, so how much time does it actually take?' Although this is just one snapshot, it represents a very common theme and it is representative of the plight of the multitude, although not generally made known to others.

On this occasion, the meeting led to our working together and I listened to her story unfold. I heard that following the birth she had been very sick and was kept in hospital for a couple of weeks. It was during this time that her baby was 'disposed' of. I use that word because she didn't know what had happened to it. Other people had attended to these details to 'save' her. My years of working in this area have shown me that this is a very common occurrence. But it left my client not ever knowing what had happened to her baby – whether it was buried or cremated, for instance, or if there had been a service. It also left her without the opportunity to say hello and good-bye to her child and to share her experience with another. She had not been allowed to hold or even see her baby and consequently did not even know whether she had a son or a daughter. 'Best not to talk about it' was the caution offered by the medical authorities of those times, and so she never did. 'Time would heal' she was assured and in the absence of anything else, this she believed. And she waited.

And so for 58 years she had lived with a snowstorm inside herself. Yes, it settled in time. And her thoughts about what might have happened or what might have been had diminished, and her feelings were tucked away and kept private. But the snowstorm was reactivated every time she saw a mum with a new-born babe, held an infant in her arms or attended a funeral. And her own grand-children were a constant reminder that more time was needed to heal. Until we met. And then we began the work of grieving.

Grieving is not about forgetting, or avoiding. It is about re-membering and letting be. However, this is painful and it is a process, not an event. And it uses up a lot of emotional energy so that you will become very, very tired. These are all good reasons why most people avoid grieving and prefer instead to rely on the myth – time will heal.

Grieving somehow never seems to get to the top of people's priority lists either. There's always something else to do that is more important, or urgent, or rewarding, or at least better than spending ages crying and feeling like nothing else on earth. I have found that it is usually only when grief manifests itself in other more noticeable ways that people are prepared to do the work associated with grieving. It may be because they are having fights and rows and arguments all the time; or perhaps they reach a point where they realise they are not happy and have not been for a long time; sometimes it's because their work performance is suffering or because their behaviour is driving their loved one away; or because they are unable to sustain a long term relationship or feel comfortable with being intimate. These are only a few examples of how grief gets incorrectly expressed when it is not attended to and we wait for time to heal.

Surviving the Snowstorm

Those who do not know about the reality of grief or our snowstorm seek to find relief from other sources. Neither pills nor alcohol are helpful. Both may afford some solace for a little while, and both also have the potential to become addictive. So does any new relationship of an intimate nature that is fostered during this period. All may help you 'feel better' because they give you a fix. None will assist your capacity to grieve, nor will they make the snowstorm go away. Remove either the pills or the alcohol or the new relationship and the snowstorm revisits with increased intensity.

I am not totally against intervention with the use of medicine. I believe it does have a place if you need to break a pattern of sleeplessness or need relief from ongoing anxiety. However, my caution is to use it sparingly and to understand that any medication is neither a panacea for grief nor a substitute for the hard work of grieving. It is an ongoing sadness and concern to me that grief education in general, and knowledge about the role of grieving in particular, are not a part of the curriculum for our medical practitioners.

Using a Model

There are many different models that attempt to describe what grief is like. The snowstorm is just one. And if it helps, then it has served its purpose. I am cautious when using such analogies because they do have limitations. There is always more than one way to understand grief. Unfortunately, what is offered as a description of how some people experience grief is all too frequently turned into a prescription of how all people should grieve.

This is what has happened to the work of Dr. Elizabeth Kubler-Ross. Over thirty years ago, she was one of the first people to systematically research death, dying and grief. She focused her initial work on dying people and described what she understood was happening for them in her model of five stages of grief. People forget that much more has been discovered about grief in the intervening years and, perhaps more importantly, that her model referred particularly to the grief of dying people. It is somewhat inappropriate and inadequate, therefore, to apply that model to the grief of the bereaved survivors.

Another potential drawback in using a model to try and describe grief, is the implication that grieving is a passive process: first this happens, then that, and then you just wait for it to be all over. Time will heal. It suggests that we are unable to help ourselves, but that is not so. Yes, grief arrives and as I have already said, it is pretty overwhelming. Yet we can do something about it. When we choose to do so, then we are involved in grieving. And that is perhaps the biggest limitation of all. Models and images only ever describe grief and attempt to illustrate what it is like. They never tell us what to do about it.

Food For Thought

When time doesn't heal, we still need to cope with life somehow. Below are some of the more common coping strategies that people adopt. Everyone uses them to some degree in their everyday living, but these coping strategies become problematic when they overshadow reality and prevent us from acknowledging our grief.

Denial
Persuading yourself that something is not so. 'Ostrich attitude'. This is useful when trying to deal with stress and grief as it acts as a buffer to the reality but can become very unhelpful if continued for any length of time.

Rationalisation
The means by which we dress what is unattractive or undesirable in new clothes and convince ourselves that all is well.

Projection
Blaming someone else for your mistakes or shortcomings. A refusal to consider your own contribution to events or reflect on your own behaviour.

Displacement
Diverting emotional emphasis from one object or person to another. For example, being angry with whoever is believed

to have caused the loss, or maybe with yourself, someone else, or God. But rather than acknowledge this and express anger directly, people instead offload onto some innocent individual as the result of some trivial misdemeanour.

Withdrawal

The person may withdraw physically, emotionally, or intellectually and resort to daydreaming and being apathetic. Sulking is a classic example of withdrawal.

Regression

Return to a state of dependency in the hope they will be protected and have their worries taken care of.

Stoicism

Usually expressed in sentiments such as 'be strong', 'coping well'. Relates to an absence of emotion. A stiff-upper-lip is the first sign of *rigor mortis*.

Personal Reflection

Consider those major events in your life that you have expected time to heal.

Become aware of those indicators which reactivate the snow-storm; for example, what are the activities, places and people that you avoid in order to prevent painful memories and feelings. List the strategies that you use in order to avoid these memories.

Event	Indicators	Coping Strategy

Summary of Key Points

- We cannot control grief by rationalising it, or by thinking positive thoughts.

- Be wary of using pills and alcohol. They will not fix grief, or make it go away.

- Grief is like the snowstorm that just arrives. We have little control over it. Grieving is the hard work we do to resolve grief and ensure the snowstorm doesn't continue to recur.

- Time alone will not heal grief. It will never just go away.

- Grieving is not about avoiding or forgetting. It is about remembering and letting be.

- We all develop coping strategies with which to survive the snowstorm phase of grief. They all have a 'use-by date' and become detrimental to us when employed beyond this time.

- The snowstorm is offered as a means to describe the onset of grief. It is not intended as a prescription of how all people 'should' experience it.

6 *Myth: You should be over it by now.*

> *Reality: There is no 'use-by date' within which to complete your grieving.*

This myth is a common refrain that is expressed primarily by people who have either not had a major loss in their lives, or who have but have not yet grieved. And as we are discovering, this process can be avoided in any number of ways: the continuing adherence to these myths being a key one. The motivating force (albeit unconscious) of these people who believe they mean well and are offering good advice is to somehow control or distance themselves from the distress and discomfort of the grieving in order, of course, to stay disconnected from their own. It is somewhat ironic that in the midst of their all-consuming snowstorm, grieving people somehow find sufficient compassion to tolerate this kind of response and frequently end up comforting the deliverer of such messages, when it is they who need to be comforted.

So people continue to offer this refrain or some other platitude such as 'Just forget it' or 'Think of the positives', 'Be strong', 'But that's not grief' or (the most commonly offered advice of all) 'Time will heal'. Despite the fact that this advice is given with the best intentions it is usually inaccurate, inappropriate and nearly always destructive – because it is delivered unconsciously, either from ignorance or inexperience. Nobody ever tells us – and we are not taught – how to deal with grief effectively. Consequently a large majority of people simply don't know how to grieve, or in fact that they need to. A person may therefore experience grief but never grieve.

Such was the case of the woman mentioned earlier whose baby was stillborn 58 years ago. She knew her business was not finished because each memory still caused her pain. But she had held fast to the advice that had been given her by those whom she believed to be appropriately qualified and knowledgeable professionals. And she had never grieved.

Nowadays we know more about grief and the process of grieving and can offer a healthier and more appropriate alternative. This is to choose to control and gain knowledge of your own grieving process. In other words, the opportunity to fully recover and get well again.

Once you understand the process and what needs to be done, you can set upon this journey in your own time and at your own pace. You can choose what, when and the length of time you wish to spend.

There are four main areas that require our attention. Grief affects us physically, intellectually, emotionally and spiritually. So not surprisingly, we need to focus our work and subsequent growth in these four areas.

Whenever we are involved with someone, or attached to something because it has significance for us, we will have invested our time, energy and feelings in that person or thing. We will have done things a certain way or have become used to things being there for us. However, we very rarely ever say this. More commonly we refer to loving something, whether it be a person, the dog, a car, a sport we play, or our job. It means that whether we care to admit it or not, we have become attached to who or what it is we love – with every dimension of our being. To a bigger or smaller degree, our thinking, feelings and personal growth will have been attached to or affected by this love. I picture it like this:

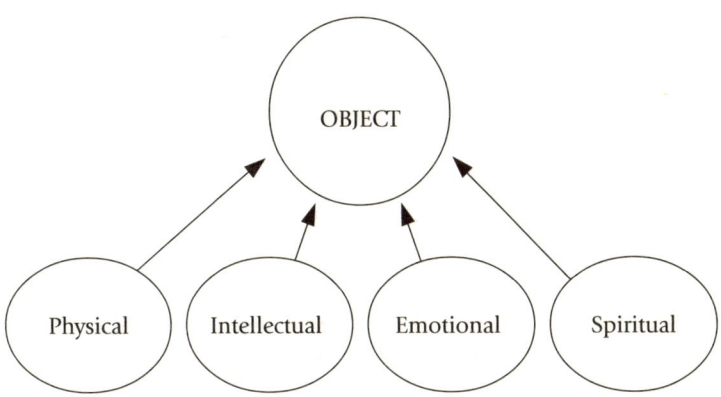

When the focus of our love is a person, the connection is stronger, and more complex because it happens both ways. Like this:

Person 1

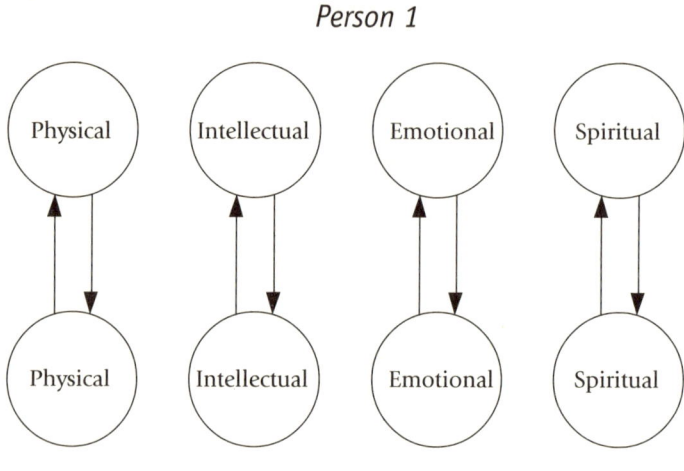

Person 2

When we lose the focus of our love, every dimension of our being has to lose its attachment to that focus. The physical disconnection is usually the most obvious and happens first, of course. Suddenly what we used to have is missing. But the well-kept secret about grief is that we need to work at disconnecting intellectually, emotionally and also spiritually from what we have lost. This is where the hard work comes in and what takes time. We need to withdraw the energy that has been expressed in our thoughts, feelings and being from what it is we have loved. And we need to do this gradually and with care.

This work is often interpreted to mistakenly mean that we can no longer have an association with what has been lost, or that we must somehow forget and leave our memories behind.

It does mean that we can no longer have the same relationship we once had. Grieving then is the work of transformation into a new, different, and more appropriate relationship in accordance with the new circumstances. There is a very big difference between hanging onto what has been and wishing it could still be, and doing this work of disconnecting and being left with wonderful, pain-free memories and a new connection that is now more realistic.

When grief is the result of death, there has often been the time and opportunity for the dying person to come to terms with their death, and they gently withdraw their energy from those they are leaving behind and begin to disconnect from them. This is what the dying process is all about. But their death and subsequent physical removal from us does not automatically mean that we have become detached from them. The connections at other levels still remain, like this:

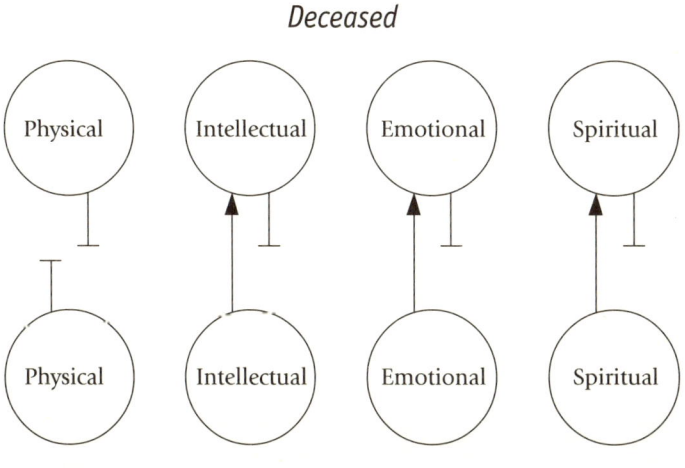

Deceased

Survivor

This is why we need to grieve – it allows us to heal from this parting. Then we can move on and continue to grow beyond that which has had its time. It is not about forgetting anything or anyone. It is about quietly letting go, in order to let be, so that we do not continue to cling to a part of life that is no longer real. In the process we learn how to have a different relationship with what has been lost.

Although the areas in which we need to focus are defined, the work required to move on in each is related to the nature of the loss, the circumstances surrounding this loss and individual need. At best I can only offer a generalised description of what is involved. The specific work of grieving is personal to you.

The work of grieving is focused on the following:

I. *Coming to believe what has happened and accepting that reality*

II. *Getting inside your feelings*

III. *Making changes and learning how to live life differently*

IV. *A spiritual quest*

PART I

Coming to Believe What has Happened and Accepting That Reality

This is the work that brings us to acceptance and involves us doing something. I think of this as the physical work.

The *Oxford Dictionary* defines acceptance as 'consent to receive; approval, belief, toleration'. It defines belief as 'acceptance of thing, fact, statement as true or existing'. So the work in this area is twofold. First, it is about doing what we need to do in order to convince ourselves that what has happened is true. This in itself takes quite a while as we fight with disbelief and struggle to rationalise that there must have been a mistake.

The second part of the task is just as difficult. When we have done everything we can do to convince ourselves that it really has happened, then we are faced with having to live with that reality. We have to 'consent to receive' it, or take it into ourselves. We may never approve of what has happened; at best we may only be able to resign ourselves to it but we do have to tolerate and learn to live with it. Resignation, however, is not full acceptance.

So, first we need to prove that what has happened is real, and then we need to accept that reality.

Many people do part of the work and get to a point where they can acknowledge what has happened. But there is a long journey from acknowledgement to acceptance. It is the difference between intellectual assent and emotional response. Acceptance is when the knowing has moved from your head to your heart. Some people never make that journey.

When we have experienced a major loss in our lives, it is very difficult to take it on board, to really believe that this has happened to us. It doesn't much matter what kind of loss either. It can be the death of a child, the loss of a job, a house destroyed by bush fire, a partner leaving the marriage or relationship, being told you have multiple sclerosis, amputation of a body part, facing life with a deformity or having a truck load of timber fall on the car. Our first response is nearly always 'This can't be true'. And then we set about to prove exactly that: it isn't true. Someone has made a mistake. We become angry and frightened. At this point there is often either panic or despair. Both are usually accompanied by tears. People repeat to us over and over again what has happened and we simply cannot take it in. We cannot believe it. We do not want to believe it. Many people have shared with me that their first response on being told of a major loss was 'You're joking!'

When the loss is related to someone dying, there is a well established and socially acceptable pattern of tasks that guide us in our initial responses. A funeral director is contacted; arrangements are made for a funeral service; a notice goes in the local newspaper to announce the death to others; arrangements are made for either burial or cremation, and then for a memorial stone or plaque to be put in place. All of these factors help make the death real. That is why the bereaved need to be involved in all aspects. It gets harder and harder to deny reality once you have sat and discussed funeral arrangements, worded a notice for the paper and attended a service.

However, other losses of major significance are afforded neither the same respect nor the social means with which to deal with them. Admittedly when the loss is caused by something other than death, considerations vary. But the work is still the same. You will need to establish the facts and gather information that will help you understand and come to terms with what has happened. You will need to fill in whatever gaps there are in either your experience or knowledge. Surprisingly, perhaps, a lot of the same sort of things can also be helpful. For example:

- When there is loss of a body part or function, having a service or ritual to acknowledge this will help increase reality and lead to acceptance. It can be a service of thanks for what has been, a committal for what has been lost, or of acceptance for the new you.

- Visiting the scene where something happened always helps to face reality, whether it is the scene of an accident, a house fire, floods, suicide, or the scene of a turbulent childhood.

- When the losses are developmental or related to child-hood, acknowledge that fact and what you missed out on. Be kind to yourself. Buy a Dr Suess book or swing in the park after dark or watch Walt Disney videos – what-ever fits for you.

- Have a burial service for your pet and keep photos of it around.

- Talk to the boss if you have been made redundant. Ask questions, not in a blaming or critical manner, but in a way that will help get the information you need to under-stand this monumental change. Persist until it has been explained in a way that you can understand because then your reality will shift. Redundancy will not be about you personally, or someone wanting to get at you; rather it might be about finances, or new machinery, or a company merger.

Take some time to reflect on what it is you want to do and then think carefully about how you might go about doing this. When will you do it? Do you want someone to be there with you, or do you want to be alone? Who do you want to be with you? Who can you tell about it? What is needed is a safe place and for you to be cared for in the process, because you will stir up emotions. Dealing with these is the focus of the next area of work, but right now you are working on giving yourself permission to do what you intuitively know is best for you, and will most help you to face and accept reality.

Fifty-eight years after the birth of her stillborn child, our mother chose to search her medical records at the hospital. She also visited the local cemetery and searched their records. She then went to the unmarked grave and placed flowers on it. In due course she approached some friends to attend a memorial service which she had planned with much love and care. And finally she had a headstone erected that announced the birth, death, and name of her daughter. And then because her husband too had been dead for some years, she went and sat on his grave and told him all she had done. At last, she was at peace.

You may choose to approach things differently but it is essential that you *do* something. The most effective task you can do, and that which will bring lasting relief and acceptance, is to talk. Talk, talk, talk. And keep talking, until you can hear the words you are saying, and believe them. And be convinced by them. You will need to talk a lot and for a long time. The same story over and over again; every little detail of it. Talking helps rewrite the computer program inside you. Every time you tell a little bit of the story you are beginning to alter the old program, and are integrating this new experience and thus creating your new reality. This is why it helps to have lots of friends and people around – the listening can be shared.

Yet this is the very thing that most people find hardest to do. 'I mustn't be a burden to my friends', 'They have heard it all before', 'Who would be interested anyway', 'I'm not sure I want them to know', 'I'm no good with words', 'They wouldn't understand', 'It doesn't matter'. Do any of these sound familiar? They are all common messages people give themselves. And they are very effective. They all prevent you from talking.

If you don't talk, your experience remains very much alive but buried. It is a secret, in the dark. It needs to be brought into the light to be made real so that you can heal. If it is left buried it will grow, usually grotesquely. Talking relieves pressure and confusion. It also reduces your isolation and feelings of aloneness. Telling your story is not about 'getting it right'. Real friends are not interested in whether the words are 'right' or 'wrong' or in your pronunciation or grammar. But they are interested in you and care about you. Let them. Avoiding or refusing to talk is not an option. It will keep you stuck in your grief and will not help you to face the reality of what has happened. Only an ostrich with its head in the sand doesn't talk.

When you begin to think about what it is you need to do, or know, ask yourself whether this will help you believe in what has happened and help you adjust. Why ask this question?

Because I want to eliminate any potential for misunderstanding. I am not suggesting that you try to get revenge, create a fantasy, avoid the issue, deny the facts or blame others. I want to help you realise your loss so that you can get on with your grieving.

One of the most precious memories I have and which still causes a great welling of emotion for me, is the mum who wanted so desperately to sing a lullaby to her little one. She had never had the opportunity to do this because her child had been aborted. In time she organised an appropriate place in which to do this, and ensured that she was surrounded by people who would support her. She then began to speak what until then had been the unspeakable, and thus began to tell her story. It led on to creating an impromptu service for her baby. And because ours was a personal friendship I held her and loved her. And we all sang 'Twinkle Twinkle Little Star' with her.

Food For Thought

Here are some suggestions of things you might do. Some of them are activities that others have shared with me. None can be classed as right, wrong, or inappropriate. All of them have been appropriate for someone. We can never dictate to anyone else what they should or should not do.

- Plant a shrub or tree.
- Erect a plaque or memorial.
- Write your own special memorial service. Invite friends to attend.
- Talk about the person who has died, or what has been lost. Continue to use the person's name.
- Choose a special candle and light it often.
- Paint, draw, sculpt, or embroider your story.
- Write about what has happened in a letter, a poem, or keep a journal.
- Make an album or a collage or some other symbol to record the event.
- Buy, or keep something special as a memento.
- Visit the place where someone died, or the scene of the loss.
- Access medical, police, and/or funeral records.
- Create a tribute or ritual.
- Ask others who were present at the event for details.
- Go through photos with family and friends.
- Join a support group.
- Go to your favourite place where you can be alone with your memories.
- Have a memories box and put all the special things into it. Visit it often.

Personal Reflection

Ask yourself these questions to help clarify what it is you need
to do to help you face what has happened

What do I want to know?

How will knowing this help me?

Who can tell me what I need to know?

How can I approach this person?

Is there anything that I haven't done that I feel I would
like to do?

Is there anywhere special I would like to go and visit?

What would help most to convince me of what has
happened?

How can I organise for this to happen?

What is it that deep down I know I really want to do,
but which I can't admit to anybody?

Is it possible to do this?

What more do I feel I would like to say to the deceased?

Who can I talk to about my experience?

PART II

Getting Inside Your Feelings

This is the emotional work of learning what you are feeling, what your feelings are telling you, what you need to do in response to them, and being able to share them with someone else.

The moment you began to carry out any of the activities that were suggested in the previous section, your emotions would have been stirred. Even if you chose to do something that was not listed, something would be happening inside of you.

The difficulty about this part of grieving is that many are unable to work out what it is they are feeling. Sometimes there are so many feelings being experienced at the same time that it is hard to name just one; mostly people are aware that they feel awful. And in other cases, people have learnt to survive by anaesthetising their feelings and have come to believe that they either don't have them or that to express them is unsanitary.

I often think that having feelings is a bit like making a milkshake. When you start to make a milkshake there are separate ingredients; milk, flavouring, thickening and ice cream. Put them altogether, mix them all up and what have you got? A milkshake. Our feelings start out as quite separate ingredients too; sadness, relief, anger, guilt, love – whatever. When we leave them unattended, they mix up inside of us and blend like an unsavoury milkshake so that they become unrecognisable. It doesn't taste good. It makes us sick.

This raises the problem of what to do with our feelings when they are stirred up, or at the very least how to make ourselves feel better. The majority of people tend to avoid intense, painful, and often embarrassing emotions. They have usually become expert at doing this in a variety of ways. And I'm now saying that not only do we need to become aware of our feelings, but that we need to let ourselves experience them fully. This is very different from just talking about our feelings, although this is a good starting point. Because as long as feelings are kept inside, all mixed up together, we cannot deal with them. We just feel confused and at a loss to understand. We need to express each feeling – to put it outside ourselves one by one. When we do, it is possible to feel each fully and deal with it. And then the next one. And the next.

The type of family system that you have been brought up in and that influenced your formative years will affect your ability to express your feelings now. Say for example that 'Let's not talk about it' was the way important issues were dealt with in your family, then it will be extremely difficult for you to now begin to talk about what is going on for you. You will be trying something that will seem foreign to you, and possibly not quite right. A need for loyalty to your family system will conflict with the work that is necessary, which is definitely to talk about and experience your feelings.

Similarly, if the family system has been about avoiding intimacy, and this means not letting others see how you feel, then you will probably be at a loss. There has been no model of behaviour for you to learn from. When this is the case, people also find it difficult to even name their feelings.

Other social systems also foster a neglect, or at best an indifference, towards our emotional development. School systems are focused on developing our intellectual abilities, and the work place still continues to make a distinction between personal and professional development. In other words, personal issues (which arouse emotions) are not seen as legitimate or relevant to the workplace. Religious systems can impose a formula of punishment and forgiveness with which to accommodate those feelings that are perceived to be socially unacceptable.

Is it any wonder then that we have difficulty in owning and expressing our feelings? There is very little in our culture that assists us to do so. Why is it that dealing with any kind of issue that may lead to confrontation or conflict with another is so widely avoided? Why is it that people adhere to the adage 'Best not to … it might upset them'. Usually it is because very strong feelings will emerge, and we don't know what do to with them.

I find that people first need to create or find an environment that is safe. In this environment they can then learn to recognise feelings, talk about them, identify the thought patterns that control them (it's not nice/lady-like/christian/adult to be angry) and finally to let them show, just a little.

Our ability to express our feelings is also related to our self-esteem. If our self-esteem is low, the thought of letting people see how we feel (by this stage usually awful) is frightening, and filled with the fear that nobody will like us. Guilt and shame often surface at this point. Guilt because others keep telling us, or we tell ourselves, that we should be over it by now, or that we shouldn't be feeling this way; and shame because we realise that we are not (over it) and no amount of effort or wishful thinking on our part seems to change how we feel. Guilt is feeling bad about what we have done. Shame is feeling bad about who we are. Learning to respect our emotions and looking after ourselves while we are experiencing them is an important part of grieving. All too frequently people try to dismiss these feelings hurriedly, or continually reproach themselves for having them in the first place.

We all have the right to have and express our feelings. We therefore need to make friends with them. Our other senses (sight, touch, smell, hearing, taste) put us in touch with the world outside ourselves. Our feelings tell us what is going on inside. They are ours. They belong to no-one else. Neither is anyone else responsible for them. Only you have power over your feelings. No other person can make you feel a particular way or tell you what to feel.

Assuming responsibility for your feelings, listening to what they are telling you and learning how to express them appropriately is what's involved in this aspect of grieving. In particular it involves experiencing and expressing those feelings you have in relation to the person who has died, or the loss you have suffered. It is not healthy or helpful to keep pushing them away or keep them hidden. This will not help you one little bit. In fact doing this will make you sick. You may have convinced yourself otherwise but knowing what you are feeling is the only way you can be in touch with yourself. It is the route to knowing who you are. Feelings are the language of the soul.

Here is an overview of common feelings encountered in grieving:

Sadness

Probably the most common feeling associated with death and loss. It is not always expressed in tears. It is often confused with depression.

Self-Reproach

This is usually felt when someone thinks they could have done something better, or could have prevented an event from happening. It can surface when they consider they were not being kind enough, or good enough.

Anxiety

The degree of anxiety can vary enormously from a feeling of insecurity to panic attacks. It usually relates to fear of an uncertain future or facing life alone. It can also be the result of becoming aware of your own vulnerability or mortality.

Loneliness

There is no longer any sense of belonging, to anyone or anywhere, and no-one to share decision making with. It feels safer often to simply stay home and not go out.

Fatigue

No matter how much you rest, or sleep, there is this continual feeling of being overwhelmingly tired. Doing anything is an effort, especially getting up in the mornings.

Helplessness

Nothing that you know or do seems to be of any use right now. It is usually present in the early stages of the snowstorm and you feel powerless to do anything about what is happening to you

Shock

Most often present in the event of sudden and/or traumatic loss and death. Can be devastating, and seems as if the world has stopped for a little while, or at least as if you are not part of it.

Yearning

Sometimes referred to as pining. A common experience that can be very intense and go on for a long time. It is often expressed by going looking for what has been lost and calling out for a loved one, or a much loved pet.

Numbness

Not feeling anything after a major loss is the way our body looks after us. It usually offers protection from a flood of feelings that could initially be overwhelming and wears off gradually as we do the work of grieving.

Anger

Anger is a God-given gift that alerts us to the fact that our rights are being violated. It is a form of self-protection. Its real purpose is to help us become more aware of ourselves and what is happening. Anger overlies hurt and when we acknowledge, accept and deal with the hurt then we can stand up for our rights and our anger will abate. Anger can be expressed constructively or destructively. The responsibility of choice is yours.

Guilt

There are two kinds of guilt. Real or culpable guilt, and imagined guilt. This is why it is so important for people to be able to express their guilty feelings and have them listened to; they need to work out, if what they are feeling, has a real basis. It is of no consequence what anybody else may think. Comparing behaviour with beliefs and values is intensely personal.

Depersonalisation

Can be experienced in a number of ways, but the most common is for people to say that they feel as if they are watching as an observer, almost as if they weren't involved or couldn't be seen. Some describe an experience of floating to the ceiling and looking down. It is a strategy we activate in order to protect ourselves from sudden and overwhelming pain.

There are of course, many more feelings that we experience. There are those we find pleasant, and those not so pleasant. Pleasant feelings are often labelled positive while the not so pleasant are usually called negative feelings. It is not wrong to have them; rather it is normal and healthy. They can arrive in a flash, or slowly. Some last a long time, some go away quickly. Sometimes several arrive simultaneously. When this happens people become confused. It is even more difficult when we have opposing feelings at the same time. But when we do not listen to our feelings and do nothing about them, they have nowhere to go – and often end up in stomach aches, headaches or bad dreams. Feelings are persistent and will bother us one way or another until we take action.

So far I have tried to raise your awareness about your feelings. But there is actually a whole process of learning involved. Moving from not allowing yourself to have any, not being aware of them or thinking them unimportant, to being able to express them adequately and appropriately takes time. The scope of this is beyond anything that I might write here. And learning *about* your emotions is not the same as learning to let yourself have them and finding out what they feel like. Sometimes we need the kind of help and learning that is offered in therapy or personal development groups to enable us to do this.

Feelings are most likely to be experienced as sensations in the body: for example, restlessness or wanting to scream. But whether we like it or not they are part and parcel of grief. Even if you have not experienced anything like it before, or are unable to put a name to what is happening, you will become more aware of them as you work through the process. These sensations are a natural and normal part of grieving. They are the ones which usually begin to abate a little given time and good friends to talk to.

When grief is experienced as the result of death or separation, grieving will involve a range of emotions which are different, and personal, and which relate specifically to the person who has died or is absent. They belong to the relationship you had and need to be attended to in order to finish that relationship.

Every relationship will have a mixture of both positive and negative feelings. It is possible to have both at the same time. This is called ambivalence. What is important in grieving is to deal with each separately. They will always be present when loss occurs because there are at least two different factors happening. When we have negative feelings it is because something has eventuated; it does not mean the absent person is negative or bad. Remember also that our feelings tell us about ourselves, not about the other person. We can for example feel relief that someone has died after a long illness, and we can also feel angry that they have left us on our own.

However, confronting the ambivalence that existed in your relationship is particularly difficult work. It will require your concentration and commitment and honesty and you may not like what you discover. The positive feelings are easy to own and express. However, if we just attend to the good side of someone who has left us, we tend to idealise that person. We make them into something perfect and cannot bear to hear any criticism that others may express. The deceased or absent person reigns from a pedestal and becomes untouchable and unapproachable as we fantasise their perfection.

If we just attend to the negative, one of two things usually happens. Either these feelings are externalised and the absentee is blamed for everything – when this occurs, the survivor becomes like a victim and is unable to acknowledge or accept any responsibility for their part in the relationship or for their feelings – or these negative feelings are internalised and the survivor becomes mute as they wither in shame for being bad enough to have these feelings in the first place.

I hope that I have conveyed that it is not only normal to have such a wide range of feelings, but allowing yourself to express them is a necessary part of grieving. Your feelings have to be felt, and only you can do that. This is the bit I cannot assist you with.

If you are at a loss over how to proceed with this work, there are people and groups who can help you. There is a vast range of literature and video material that is designed to help people carry out emotional work. Alternatively, good friends will be invaluable during this phase of grieving. Be discerning about who you choose to share your feelings with. Ultimately the listener who will be most helpful will be someone who is non-judgemental, accepting of who you are, able to hear the bad as well as the good, and not afraid of any feelings you might want to express. And rather than wanting to calm your 'upsetness' they will ensure your safety and respect your confidence.

Food for Thought

Here are some more suggestions of practical things you can do to assist the emotional work.

- Respect your own feelings.
- Allow yourself to cry.
- Check your progress periodically. For example are the down times less frequent or less intense than they were originally?
- Listen to music, dance, sing, play an instrument.
- Share your experience with other people: talk to a friend, join a support group, go to a counsellor or someone who is a trained listener.
- Find an isolated spot and scream.
- Wear an article of clothing that belonged to the absent person.
- Carry a memento.
- Express how you feel, with paints, poetry, writing or sculpting.
- Hug a teddy bear or soft toy. Pat a pet.
- Learn how to express anger constructively.
- Write yourself a letter of love, or forgiveness.
- Write a letter to the person who is absent and read it out loud.
- Sit and talk to a photograph of your loved one. Tell them how it is for you now.

Personal Reflection

Here are a few thoughts that will help stimulate your emotional awareness. There are no 'right' or 'wrong' answers, though some indicate a healthier state of development than others. Answer the questions Never, Sometimes, Often.

	N	S	O
Do you feel you have to hide your real feelings?			
Are you able to show affection freely?			
Do you think it is good for adults to cry?			
Are you embarrassed to have anyone see you cry?			
Do you feel intimidated when someone expresses anger?			
Are you able to express anger?			
Do you find it hard to let people get close to you?			
Are you afraid your feelings will get hurt easily?			
Do you worry what others think of you?			
Are you able to laugh at yourself?			
Do you feel you have choices in circumstances?			
Are you able to be playful?			
Do you like to feel people need you?			
Are you afraid of upsetting people?			
Do you respond to both physical and emotional pain?			
Are you aware of what your body is feeling?			

Practise naming your feelings.

Draw up a chart and record which ones you experience most often.

PART III

Making Changes and Learning How to Live Life Differently

This is the intellectual work of problem-solving, decision making and learning new skills and 'know-how' in order to adjust and survive without what it is you have lost.

The nature of the loss and the importance of it will influence the work that is done here. New skills may have to be learned, your belief systems may need to be reviewed or you may have to alter some routine. But continuing to live life as if nothing has happened, or as if there has been no change, is simply a form of denial. Some form of adjustment to the way you live your life is always necessary if you are to move forward and heal from your grief.

Sometimes the adjustment required is obvious; sometimes it is more subtle. Our awareness of the need for adjustment usually awakens slowly, often in response to other events. Sometimes there are several adjustments to be made. Mostly however, they require a lot of thought and reflection and at times investigation before people are ready to make changes.

This part of grieving is concerned with problem-solving and largely occupies the intellectual part of ourselves as we struggle to attain independence again in the face of our loss. First we have to identify what it is we need to learn or deal with and then discover how to do it. This can be illustrated by giving an example of what might be involved when a partnership has ended. Whether this is by death or separation is irrelevant; one or each partner will now have to adjust to living on their own.

In most partnerships, the workload will have been shared. There will have been some tasks that each assumed quite naturally, or have agreed to divvy up. This varies with different generations of course and from couple to couple – but I have found that because of their skills or time commitments or interest in a particular area, each person in a partnership will tend to take on different responsibilities.

When one person dies or leaves the partnership, the other is left often not knowing how to undertake the tasks that their partner did. They may have looked after the finances and managed all the bookwork. If the remaining partner has never had to worry about balancing a chequebook, working to a budget, or paying the bills, then the fact that they now have to may be frightening. They will have no idea of where to start or how to go about organising it.

Obviously I am not making this point in order to criticise a lack of bookkeeping skills or to cast judgement about whether everyone should keep their own finances. My point is that a new task has to be learned in order for the partner to be independent. Unless they learn about chequebooks and bank statements and develop some system that enables them to pay their bills on time, they will forever be in trouble and life will be stressful. Unfortunately what happens all too frequently is that people are unable to refrain from casting aspersions on the person who asks for help. Admitting that they don't know how to do their banking is daunting enough – having to experience shame as well because of a comment that conveys the message, 'Good heavens, you're how old, and you don't know how to do this?' is soul destroying. If it is necessary to say anything, it is more appropriate to acknowledge that they haven't had either the need or opportunity to learn this skill earlier, and isn't it wonderful that they have the courage and determination to do so now in order to retain their independence.

There are many changes in routine that people experience when a relationship ends. Perhaps cooking (and other domestic chores) were one partner's responsibility. Should the cook die, or leave the relationship, the remaining partner will need to develop cooking skills. Where do you learn to do this? Particularly, where do you learn at a later stage in life? All too often it is taken for granted that cooking is something everyone can do. But if you have never been taught and never had to do it, then what? Some may adapt quite easily. Trial and error may improve their efforts over time. But for others it may well appear to be a task that is beyond their capabilities – and both their health and their social life will suffer as a result.

The issues are usually different, but what is common to all is the need to think about and plan how to accomplish tasks that were taken for granted.

Although I have illustrated this point by discussing issues surrounding the loss of a partner (either by death or separation), the themes raised are common following most losses. In order to adjust to the change in their lives, people find they have to begin to think about who they are, how they want to refit into the world again, how they can feel safe about doing this and how they can feel good about themselves as they do so.

Every effort in this process is about regaining or retaining whatever measure of independence is possible. The specific adjustments each individual makes will be different and reflect the particular loss experienced, but consider the following:

- Loss of mobility following a stroke may require thinking about home help, having a live-in companion, or leaving home and going to an institution where full-time care is available.

- Loss of good health may result in a person being confined to their home more, and may require thinking about how to retain social contact they had previously enjoyed: e.g. at bowls, choir etc.

- Job loss means a drastic alteration to the finances. Getting another job may not be easy and finances may be restricted for some time. Questions to consider might include; do you keep the mortgage going, sell the house, take in lodgers, rent it out and stay with friends, increase the mortgage to tide you over, or give up any thought of working again and adjust to being a beneficiary?

- Promotion may require some changes: more socialising, more study, longer hours of work, change of friends. And how is this to be balanced with a growing family and their needs for your participation?

- Loss of a body part has an impact on a person's self-image and confidence. How is the hygiene and odour of a colostomy to be managed in social settings? How to put the rubbish out now that you are in a back brace and unable to lift anything heavy? The reason for the loss will also be a separate issue in itself that people will need to face and adjust to.

- People in wheelchairs, whatever their state of health, are faced with making monumental changes in their lives and lifestyles, as well as being faced daily with the practical challenges of how to enter buildings, open heavy doors, drive a vehicle, have a bath.

- Loss of a home immediately presents the problem of where to find warmth, food, shelter and clothing. It raises many more issues to be addressed in the longer term.

After a significant loss, some people adjust quite quickly, while for others it is a long, slow process. And while the need for change is being grappled with, life goes on. Maybe you still have to go to work, the children still need to be attended to, you still have to shop and cook and wash and iron and get the car fixed and the cat to the vet and go to a friend's wedding, or deal with the death of a family member. This is what makes life seem so unfair – it just keeps on keeping on. Life presents yet more for you to cope with and yet you are still struggling with the initial loss and adjustments required as a result.

Because of your vulnerability during this time, other people quite naturally want to help. And because of your exhaustion, you tend to let them. Frequently however, these same people are not aware of boundaries and their well intentioned efforts turn into taking over, or trying to control your life by making decisions for you. If this happens, 'caring for you' turns into something more controlling and potentially destructive – an action I call 'care-taking', as in a sense, genuine caring has been taken away, rather than given. (See further discussion in Chapter 10.) The prospect of making major or new life decisions can be daunting and you may find yourself shying away from it. But as long as you are unable to make decisions on your own you will be dependent on others, and usually they do not carry out what you would have wanted, or would have done for yourself. So become aware of what might be preventing you from making your own decisions.

Fear is a factor that might inhibit your decision-making. Fear of getting it wrong, fear of the consequences, fear of upsetting others, fear of what 'they' might think, or say. Other factors may include not wanting to go against the known or imagined wishes of the deceased. Unfortunately these fears will keep you stuck or restricted. They are also very personal and given time and the support of caring friends or a counsellor, they can be addressed, and some freedom then gained to make your own decisions.

However, there is another aspect which gets raised time and again and which seems common to many. It is the belief that having made a decision, it cannot be changed. I am appalled by this credo now, although there was a time in my life when I did subscribe to it. It is reinforced by many clichés that are quoted unthinkingly: 'You've made your bed, now you have to lie on it'; 'What's done is done and can't be undone'; 'It's God's will'; 'Life's a bitch'; 'You'll never be given more to cope with than you can bear'. All such sayings that leave us powerless and imply that this is how life is. All we can do is grin and bear it. Or...

Or, you could make another decision. It may require a study of your own beliefs: where have these messages come from? What exactly do they mean, why do I accept them, who would I offend if I did not accept them? These are all questions you may need to ask before you feel free enough to make another decision. It may also require you to face the fact that you are not superwoman or superman, or indeed perfect, and that you may have made a mistake. Again, what you believe about mistakes will affect how you feel about changing your mind. One school of thought considers mistakes to be bad, wrong, a sign of imperfection, and something that should be punished. At the other end of the continuum is the point of view that mistakes are the best way to learn. Making mistakes is a means to making corrections, discovering our humanity, improving performance and something that can be shared and discussed. Where do you fit on this continuum?

Maybe it's time to reconsider and adopt different beliefs. My view is that we make a decision in any given moment with what information is to hand and on the basis of our experience. Any or all of these three components will change: the circumstances, information available and our experience. In light of this, it seems realistic to keep making decisions that reflect our current situation. Our decisions are not set in concrete to be worshipped for all time. We simply make the best decision we can at the time we make it. And then keep checking it out and seeing if the effects of that decision are what we planned or wanted.

If making decisions on our own is something new to you, doing so now will feel strange. You may not be clear about what it is you want. But start making little decisions by yourself, and for yourself. Hold to them in the face of opposition. By doing this you will retain control of your life and discover what you want.

There are also many personal issues to be considered when

you begin to socialise again. The trouble with grief and grieving is that there are no crutches or bandages that give an indication to others. It is therefore unreal to expect people to look after you. This is part of the adjustment you will need to make for yourself. Other people are always keen for you to socialise very quickly after a loss, and may pressure you to do so. They see it as a return to normality.

But usually it takes some time before you will be ready. If, for example, you have lost a partner through death or separation, it is as if you have lost half yourself, and without the benefit of anaesthetic. Of course you will nurse yourself carefully and not want to go places where your wound might possibly get knocked. You will not be keen either to be seen and will want to wait until healing is well advanced before socialising. Grieving people all carry a wound. The extent is related to the size of the loss, but always they are presented with the question of how to re-engage socially following the loss or crisis.

Do you talk about the loss, or wait for someone else to mention it? Do you still wear your wedding ring after your partner dies? What name do you want to be known by now that you have separated? How do you want your friends to treat you now that you are in a wheelchair: do they push your chair, walk alongside, or help when the wheels get stuck? Now that the children have left home and you are returning to work, how do you wish to be addressed – by name or by title? How do you socialise as an older single in a couples oriented society?

This is the work of redefining who you are in light of what has happened. You may continue as if nothing has happened, but that's unreal, difficult for your friends, and likely to lead to a snowstorm at any time. And when nothing gets talked about, it is like having an elephant in the room that has to be stepped around while nobody acknowledges the great pile of dung it has just deposited.

This playing pretend, or continuing to adhere to family or social rituals as if everything is still the same, is something I would encourage you to reconsider. Christmas, birthdays, anniversaries, are all potent times that remind us of our loss. 'This time last year I was…'. So many people wait in fear for such occasions and feel powerless in the face of them. I'd encourage people not to shrink from them, but to plan in advance. Give careful thought to where you want to be, who you'd like to be with, and how you want to mark these days. And if you choose to be on your own with a picnic in the woods rather than at the traditional Christmas dinner, then tell people and ask them to respect your decision.

Remember: life is different now, and so are your needs. Make your changes accordingly, rather than clinging to a past that is no longer real.

Food For Thought

Some practical suggestions for this phase of grieving.

- Allow yourself time to adjust. This is a lengthy and ongoing process that will not be resolved in a matter of weeks or months.
- When someone offers to help you with something – let them.
- Do what feels right for you, not what other people say you 'should'.
- Avoid making hasty decisions, especially major ones like moving house.
- Have a plan for each day. One task, one day at a time.
- Plan ahead and decide how you want to spend anniversaries, weekends, holidays.
- Develop new skills in community classes.
- Learn to identify what it is you need and develop the assertiveness to ask for it.
- Ask others what adjustments they have made to cope with loss.

Personal Reflection

The following questions may be of value as you assess any given situation when trying to decide whether or not to make changes.

What do I gain from not changing?

Would I be willing to give up any of the above gains I have identified? State which ones.

What do I gain by changing?

Do the gains of not changing outweigh the gains of changing?

If so, why?

If not, am I willing to make the change?

Can I enlist the support, understanding and co-operation of others?

What are my short-term goals?

What are my long-term goals?

What changes will help me achieve these goals?

PART IV

A Spiritual Quest

This is about searching for a life philosophy or frame-work within which you can make sense of what has happened. It will provide meaning and purpose for you to choose to engage again with life and living.

Saying yes to living fully again is something that most force themselves to do prematurely. Often people will demand it of them, because of course, 'You should be over it by now'. But this process cannot be forced. It is the fruit of all the hard and painful work of attending to your grief. A flicker of interest that draws you back into the mainstream is the first sign of healing. This is the beginning of the end of a natural, normal process. It saddens me to know that all too frequently it is not allowed to run its course. There is no set time-frame, and it is dependent on whether the grieving (associated with the three previous tasks) has been attended to. Many people attempt to become involved without doing this work, and their efforts are always unsuccessful. Their thinking becomes warped because too many issues remain unaddressed. Their concealed feelings scream silently in their bodies, and their previous behaviour continues without any allowances for the differences of their current situations.

So, just as we need to grieve, there comes a time when we also need to stop grieving. One of the things which affects our ability to do so is what we have decided about what has happened to us. This requires us to think about loss and death, and what happens after death. Exploring these issues is a personal and sometimes private journey. Not many feel free to share their thinking when it comes to God or the metaphysical or the realms of the spiritual. The answers we each come to will be as diverse as we are. However, it is here, more than in any other task of grieving, that people encounter the strongly held beliefs of others that emphasise what is right and what is wrong.

Reflecting on loss, death and why someone has died will raise all sorts of questions. Why has this happened; why has it happened now; why has it happened to me; why is Bill still alive at 97 when my child died at six months; why has our family had three deaths (or accidents) in six months and others have not yet experienced any; why, why, why?

Asking 'why' begins the search that promotes spiritual growth. 'Why' gives expression to our desire to understand how this universe works and seeks to find meaning, purpose, and some acceptable order behind what has happened. 'Why' is our yearning to find some solution that is beyond any personal rationale for which we may feel responsible.

Who rules the world, is there a higher power in charge of everything and everyone, are we punished, or redeemed or just loved? Are we on our own or are we part of a co-operative venture that is transpersonal and cosmic? Is there life after death, do we have more than one go at life, what makes it all worthwhile, why is there so much pain and suffering and if there is a God why does he, she, or it, let it happen?

Many of us don't even begin to think about these issues until we are faced with a crisis. Suddenly everything seems unfair and death itself seems the biggest betrayal of the lot.

Despite its constant presence as a neighbour, we are surprised when it turns to say 'hello'.

Our answers to these questions will be endless. And in my opinion, there is no right or wrong. What is more important is that each of us ask our questions and wrestle with the pain, the unknowing, and our god in order to find our own answers. This is the last important piece in the jigsaw puzzle.

It is important, because you will then live with your philosophy, and it in turn will begin to shape your life. That is why it is also important to take care in searching for it. Whatever you decide needs to sit comfortably within you and be a source of both peace and inspiration.

You may revisit the questions and review your answers during your life or after other major life events, but until they bring you a sense of being united with yourself they will serve only to be a source of dis-ease to you.

This is not the work of the intellect – rather it is the work of the soul. It is done in an attempt to put your loss in context and to look at the bigger picture of how the world works. It is about formulating your own personalised map of life, and what is important for you in terms of values and beliefs. It is not about analysing, moralising, or justifying. But is has a lot to do with developing a faith that will keep you anchored during a storm and which enables you to trust the process of life and give up the need to control. It also has a lot to do with loving.

Many people find their answers provided in the teachings of religions. Others find these formalised answers restrictive, nonsensical, or simply unpalatable. A person does not need to be religious in order to find and give expression to their spirituality, although many would have us believe differently. The important thing is to take time to listen and consider the matters of the soul. Until you do, you will be living without this most essential part of yourself and life will never make sense. It will forever feel as if something is missing.

Your 'yes' to life and living will only come when you have allowed yourself to fully express and reflect on all the questions that arise for you. Once you have arrived at some sense of personal resolution over what life and death are all about, then you'll be able to move on from the loss you have sustained.

After experiencing the death of a loved one, you will be unable to move on until you have done this – because you'll have no beliefs about what has happened to the deceased. Will they float into nothingness, will you forget them and not be able to remember anything of what you shared, will they be at peace or will they be judged and punished? Anyone who has fears or doubts about this part of the process will be unwilling to commit the spirit of their loved one to an entity or concept whom they don't know and don't trust. Or to something they themselves don't fully accept. And while they are unable to do this, they are prevented from being able to move on because they are still enmeshed with the deceased.

This evaluation of life and of death takes quite some time. Many people try to avoid the hard questions that are presented in this part of grieving. They dismiss it cynically as 'naval gazing' or refer to it fatalistically as 'what will be will be'. And it is very easy to simply say 'I don't know' and give up and stay stuck. However, doing this work and facing the issues is essential in order to resolve your grief and is the route to growing spiritually. Spiritual awareness is a reflection of self-actualisation.

There comes the time when you need to keep moving and

living and growing. Take the learning and the love and the memories of what has been lost with you as you begin to live your life again and reach out to others. You have a lot of living and loving still to do. And doing this does not mean that you love your dead any less.

You will always love them. Now, however, you are exploring how to express that love in a different way. You are also learning how to recognise their love as it is shown to you in a new dimension: the spiritual. I suggest you read widely from the vast number of books that are now available and which address this topic more fully than I am able to here.

The work I've described in this section is what determines how you will continue to live your life. Do you choose to proceed as an embittered person who is full of regrets, anger or wanting revenge for what has happened to you? Or have you touched your soul and found some greater paradigm of understanding, within which to accommodate your loss? Your choice will bring very different results. If you choose to remain embittered, you will experience loss as a personal attack, and will feel the need to right the wrong. The other choice, however, will lead you to healing and wholeness, with the capacity of empathy for others.

Food for Thought

Here are some more ideas to help with your spiritual phase of grieving.

- Go at your own pace – there is no rigid timetable to follow nor are there stages that you 'should' go through.
- Don't expect too much and don't be too hard on yourself.
- Do something nice for yourself each day: ring a friend, have a rest, develop a hobby, soak in a bath, smell the roses.
- Take care that you eat well and are getting adequate sleep.
- Recall and acknowledge the high points, the happy memories from the past. Acknowledge also the not-so-happy and difficult memories.
- Be open to expanding your thinking and trying new things.
- Ask others to share their spiritual journeys.
- Do drive more carefully and be more careful around the home. Accidents are more common after severe loss.
- Try new experiences – yoga, meditation, T'ai Chi. Read widely.
- Take time to think and pray. It is medicine for the mind and soothing to the soul.
- Practise or learn the skill of creative visualisation.

Personal Reflection

Here are some questions to serve as beginning guidelines in spiritual self-analysis.

How would you describe the 'real' you?

What part of you do you allow others to see?

What does death mean to you?

What do you believe happens after death?

What is it that gives meaning and purpose to your life?

Where do you receive most inspiration from?

What would you describe as your God?

What is your relationship with your God?

What are your most meaningful relationships? And why?

Do you tend to your own needs? If not, why not?

How do you forgive others?

How do you define success?

Summary

I hope that now, with a more comprehensive understanding of what grieving involves, you'll see that nobody else can determine when another individual 'should be over it'.

The work I've discussed will take a different period of time for everyone. For some it will be brief; while for others it may take years. Some will do their grieving at the time of the loss; for a variety of reasons others will not complete it until years later. For some it will be an intense experience. Others will find that with the understanding and non-judgemental support of caring friends they will move through it naturally.

The work of grieving has been likened to peeling an onion. You remove one layer, only to discover that several layers underneath also have to come away. This requires you to do more work, or maybe the same work at a deeper level. And so the layers are removed until you embrace the core.

This work involves confronting not only what has happened, but adjusting to live with the changes it brings. It requires that you ask the hard questions of life and keep asking them until the search brings you to an internal peace and understanding.

You will know when you have arrived, or when this work is done. You will lose the overwhelming intensity of feeling that causes your heart to lurch whenever you are reminded of what has happened. The pain will lessen and eventually go away. You will be able to remember without dissolving into tears and feeling angry or wanting revenge. You will be able to think about it all with some degree of acceptance. You will discover an interest in living again. And the time will come when you don't have to remember. Your experience will be part of you and who you are. But it will not dominate your life and what you do and how you feel. You will also have grown in physical well-being, intellectual understanding, emotional capacity and spiritual awareness.

Grief is the price of love. Whatever we love we risk. Love for someone or something, means that if you lose it, you will be hurt... The moment we find either [happiness or love] we risk losing it, and so we risk the grief that must come with the loss.
Merren Parker, A Time to Grieve

What does achieving recovery mean? It means once again being able to do some perfectly ordinary things. Being able to feel good if something good happens. Being able to be hopeful about the future. Being able to give attention to everyday life... Being able to feel at peace with yourself.
Francis Macnab, Life After Loss

Blessed are they who mourn, for they shall be comforted.
Matt. 5:4

Sorrow, like a river, must be given vent, lest it erode the bank.
Barbara Ward, Mexican Proverb in Healing Grief

Your joy is your sorrow unmasked...
The deeper that sorrow carves into your being, the more joy you can contain...
When you are sorrowful, look [...] in your heart, and you shall see that in truth you are weeping for that which has been your delight.
Kahlil Gibran, The Prophet

Summary of Key Points

- Grieving is not a passive process. It will require action.

- The action you take will be personal and have special meaning. It will enable you to complete unfinished business and assist you to disconnect from who or what has been lost.

- What you do has much to do with your needs. It is not about seeking punishment, revenge or in any way harming another.

- The work of grieving will require you to be honest with yourself. It will also take time and energy to complete.

- The support of selected friends or a trained listener will be most helpful to assist you through this process.

- The work of grieving is a little like peeling an onion. There are many layers that need to be peeled off, or attended to.

- Resignation is very different from acceptance.

- The process of recovery is linked directly to acceptance of the loss. Acceptance cannot come until the reality of the situation is faced.

7 *Myth:* You never really get over it.

Reality: Grieving is the means by which we heal. We can recover fully from the impact of any loss.

Blockages

Those people who offer the refrain at the head of this chapter are speaking their truth. They have never recovered from their loss and grief. And so they accept this myth as truth, and use it to comfort themselves and others. Yet this saying is an indication that the speaker's grieving process is as yet unresolved or has become blocked.

We have already discussed several reasons why people may not have been able to resolve their grief. Here is a summary:

- Grieving is believed to be a passive process (time will heal)
- Myths are accepted as fact and believed unquestioningly
- The difference between grief and grieving is not appreciated
- The work of the grieving process is not well-known or understood

- Social taboos still surround some losses and thus prevent grieving
- A lack of personal growth results in limited 'response ability', in a physical, intellectual, emotional and spiritual way
- The loss has not been recognised and this has resulted in the grief becoming disenfranchised
- People choose to live with their grief rather than engage in a process that might assist them to resolve it (e.g. therapy, support group)
- The family system for dealing with grief is adopted

So when I hear anyone saying 'You never really get over it' I believe what they are saying, and know that they have never completed their grieving. Somewhere, somehow, their own grieving has been blocked. I also experience a sadness, not only for them, but for all those on whom they foist this myth and who will come to accept it as reality.

There are a number of quite common responses and behaviours that obstruct grieving. These obstructions can be self-imposed or come about from the interventions of others.

PART I

How Acceptance can be Blocked

A key way in which we block acceptance is to minimise a situation. Minimising is how we trivialise or make less of an event. When we try to reduce the impact of an event, we are being less than honest. It is the most common occurrence that prevents our moving toward full acceptance and completion of the task of grieving.

Minimising is carried out in a seemingly endless variety of ways, most of which spring to mind unconsciously. It is present in placating remarks, and in our own thinking as we constantly remind ourselves that there is always someone worse off than we are. The words people use to describe what has happened is another way of minimising a situation. You only need to think about the different words used to refer to death, without actually having to mention the word:

- 'Losing' someone
- Sleeping
- Kicked the bucket
- Pushing up daisies
- Moved on
- Passed over
- Six feet under
- Gone
- Taken from us
- No longer with us

Whether it is done deliberately or unconsciously, minimising is a form of denial that makes things appear different or not quite as bad as they seem. Without exception, it undermines either the facts, the significance or the irreversibility of any loss. And given that the amount of our grief equates with the intensity of our loss, this is a powerful means with which to reduce the loss and its impact. It may help us feel better in the short-term, but any form of minimising blocks the grieving process and keeps people stuck.

Minimising the Facts

When the facts surrounding the loss are minimised it means that in some way we do not acknowledge everything that has happened, or that we alter the facts slightly to make it more acceptable. Suicide is a classic example. As it still carries a social stigma and is not openly acknowledged, the bereaved frequently experience some shame. Unless, that is, there is sufficient reason for the media to get hold of it, in which case it is usually sensationalised. More commonly the word 'suddenly' appears in a death notice and only oblique reference is made to it at the funeral service. I have worked with many people over the years, all of whom had become stuck in their grieving as the result of not being able to openly acknowledge that a close family member had suicided. Some reported that they had found the body of the deceased and altered the environment to cause confusion and/or make it less obvious that death had been the result of suicide. Others had for years told a different story that although plausible, was untrue.

When the facts are altered, reality is being distorted, and consequently grief also becomes distorted. And there are many occasions when any alteration seems preferable to reality. Take the case of the client whose relative had 'died' while they were working overseas. After this client and I had worked together for some time, he was able to speak the truth that he had concealed for over forty years. His relative had not just died, but had been cannibalised. Although the pain associated with this reality was devastating, it was only when it was acknowledged that he could proceed with his grieving and healing ensue. Initially the minimising of this event had occurred to evade the melodramatic responses of others on hearing the news.

But over the years it had superseded reality. And as a result his grieving had been blocked.

Minimising the impact of certain situations is adopted to manage grief that is considered to be socially unspeakable. Abortion, miscarriage and the grief of those who share a same-sex relationship are examples of grief that is socially unacceptable. More often than not homosexual relationships are not approved by our society, and scant regard is given to any grief they might experience. So in order for a partner to acknowledge affiliation with the deceased, and thus have permission to grieve, the identity of the deceased is frequently altered to that of a friend or sibling. Their love can't be acknowledged; and neither can the fullness of their grief. But that does not make it any less real. And so a relationship that has been precious and wonderful and a major part of their life is minimised. And so too is their ability and opportunity to grieve.

Minimising the Significance

Minimising the importance of a loss can be done oh, so easily. 'It was only', they say. Or 'You can always get another'. 'How old was your grandmother? Oh, 93, well, she had a good long life then.' And have you noticed that if you have a broken leg (have had an operation, lost your job, had a car smash, house been burgled) someone is sure to tell you about someone they know who has had two broken legs (a bigger operation, made a career of being made redundant, survived umpteem car smashes, had several burglaries). All of these responses have the same effect for the grieving person. It stops them talking and reduces their loss, their grief, to lesser importance or to insignificance in the face of this other tale of woe. They end up feeling guilty. The message they have received has been clear; their loss doesn't warrant discussion.

And when you give yourself the same messages, the effect is exactly the same. You will fall into the trap of comparing your loss and grief to that of others and it will stop you moving forward with your own grieving. Grief cannot be compared. There is only ever your loss and how important that is for you, and another person and how important their loss is to them. And just because grandmother has lived 93 years does not mean that you are not allowed to grieve her dying. It means you have had a longer time than most with which to enjoy her life and that consequently you will miss her the more for it.

Admittedly people say these things to try and make you feel better, possibly even to help you 'think of the positives'. Or is it to make themselves feel better by having something to say? Albeit said with the best of intentions, the effect of these clichés is always damaging, as they interfere with the expression of grief. You are not ready yet to look on the bright side of things; you are struggling to look at reality. Once that is faced, then the brighter side will emerge.

Prepare a few stock rebuttals to have up your sleeve for when you encounter these types of responses. For example: 'Yes, she did have a long life. She has always been part of my life. I don't know quite what it is going to be like now without her.' 'I'm not sure I will ever want to get another. I am still hurting about losing this one.' 'I realise this may not seem important to you but it is to me. Please don't dismiss it so readily.' And when all else fails: 'I'm not ready to play Pollyanna right now. You don't have to say anything. Just stay here with me and be my friend.' Any response that states your truth will be effective, as opposed to a rejoinder that is sarcastic or belittling. The least helpful is to use another cliché.

Minimising the Irreversibility

This has to do with trying to preserve the past and what might have been. The focus is on believing that everything will come right, and things will soon be back to normal, the way they always were. When people engage in this type of behaviour, they live in a fantasy world that is created from unrealistic hope and denial. There is for example, a very natural period of time following a death or loss, where we attempt to preserve things as they were. It is normal in the short term to leave a person's room the way it was and to treasure mementoes. It is not normal to preserve something for when that person returns. Neither is it normal or helpful to continue with old behaviour like laying someone's clothes out or setting their place at the table so it will be ready for when they come back.

Some of these actions may be habitual and will therefore be done automatically after a crisis, simply because it takes a while to remember to stop doing them. I am not talking about that. I am talking about when these actions are done deliberately to await someone's return or to prove to the world that nothing has happened. It may help reduce the intensity of the loss to think that someone is going to return, or that things will return to 'normal'. But it hinders any acceptance of what has happened. It seeks to deny the reality that what has been lost cannot be reversed. When the loss involves possessions, eventually these can be replaced or restored. Unfortunately this replacement behaviour cannot reverse death. All too commonly however, people transfer this replacement behaviour as a means to cope.

Summary of Part I

When grieving is hindered by minimising an event, or any other means, the result is denial. Denial in itself is not a bad or incorrect response. However it is like consumables: it has a use-by date after which it becomes unpalatable. Denial is regularly our initial response to a crisis, and can be the very thing that enables us to survive it. Denial also becomes an inevitable alternative when there is insufficient information or an adequate explanation to help people understand what has happened. Denial results when we have been unable to tell our personal story or truth and express ourselves fully in the way that we need to. And denial arises as a consequence of not knowing how to proceed with the emotional work of grieving. But to prolong denial in the face of reality is always destructive. It prevents a person from moving on and growing, as they are then obliged to alter all future experiences to fit their warped or limited perception.

Denial is the opposite of acceptance. Minimising situations contribute toward denial. Facing any reality produces an emotional response and until the individual has the skills and support necessary to express these feelings, denial is used as a coping mechanism to keep them distant.

I have frequently been implored by people to 'shift them out of denial'. But I never attempt to force anyone out of denial. Rather I respect it, because it has a purpose and there will be a reason why a person has been compelled to employ it. When a client is ready and willing to move from denial and face their reality, we work together to identify what has caused grieving to become blocked at this point. Then we set about to rectify the block and to face reality.

PART II

Getting Inside Your Feelings:
When Emotions Are Blocked

For a variety of reasons, many people are frightened when they begin this emotional work. It can be very painful, and often the intensity of their feelings can be overwhelming. For this is the work that brings out all of those feelings that have been stored, or left unacknowledged over the years. Some individuals may have survived traumatic situations as children by freezing their capacity to feel anything. The work of thawing frozen feelings is arduous and any feeling that is unfamiliar is experienced as strange. This emotional work is therefore undertaken little by little as the client is ready, and can take some time to complete.

While you are struggling to deal with your feelings, there will be another part of you that will be struggling equally hard not to deal with them. This is a natural internal conflict that manifests itself in one of several ways. All have the effect of blocking this work and preventing grieving.

Rationalisation and Avoidance

One of the main ways we convince ourselves not to deal with feelings is by rationalising the circumstances. Our head gives us some pretty powerful messages and is persistent about why we should not do this emotional work. Some of its messages might go like this:

- You must have only nice thoughts now that the person is dead

- You must be strong for Mum (the kids, the family, everyone)
- It is wrong to have 'negative' feelings about what has happened
- You are selfish and uncaring to think about yourself at a time like this
- No-one will like you if you show them what you are really feeling
- This work is really totally unnecessary
- You must not get UPSET
- If you let your feelings out you will lose control
- You haven't the time to go into feelings right now.

Rationalising is a major block to completing this aspect of grieving. It will keep you away from painful thoughts, and from your feelings – which of course is its primary purpose. Its messages are powerful, subtle and insistent. As far as your head is concerned, any argument it can conceive that allows you to stay in control is acceptable. The irony is that irrespective of how illogical the message is, we can rationalise it until we believe it and thus convince ourselves of its authenticity.

Rationalising a situation is primarily the process by which we give ourselves messages about our behaviour. Others also do this for us, and are usually quick to endorse our explanations. This endorsement by others is a subtle conspiracy to avoid upsetting anyone. Society by and large is uncomfortable with grief and with the expression of feelings. To upset anyone is something that must be avoided at all costs. If a person has not already rationalised away their feelings, others will convey messages that have the same effect. 'Isn't she coping well' they say; or 'He's being very strong'. Which says nothing really, except to note that there is an apparent absence of emotion (or upsetness). And in light of such praiseworthy comment, those grieving dare not renege with a change in behaviour.

We all need to be upset following any major loss in our lives. I can think of no better reason to be upset. But being upset, and being socially acceptable, do not go together. And the majority of people still believe that they are responsible for other people's feelings and the fact that someone becomes upset in response to something they might have said or done. So anything that might be a reminder of the loss is avoided and any possible display of emotion is circumvented. When faced with a difficult decision or task that will stir memories, many people will rush in to 'save' the grieving from becoming 'upset'.

Rationalising our feelings is an attempt to control them. It is a means to avoid or deny or displace the pain that we don't know how to handle. However there is no other way to deal with pain than to deal with pain. In trying to remove it one way, you will simply have to face it another way, because it cannot be removed without our feeling it. Grieving is not about forgetting. Rather it is about remembering and letting be. And that is always painful.

If those around you become 'upset' when you are in touch with your feelings, then find another place and other people with whom you can express your feelings. Avoiding or denying your emotions in order to make someone else comfortable will make you sick and keep you stuck in your grief. You will not be helping yourself, and neither will you be helping them. They obviously have their own business to finish and feelings to attend to. If you look after their feelings it will prevent them from getting on and doing this for themselves.

Shifting and Keeping Busy

Another way of avoiding or delaying this aspect of grieving is to keep moving away from your feelings. And I mean this quite literally. People shift. They shift house; they shift jobs; they shift towns; they shift relationships; they shift whatever they can but the most important thing is to keep on the move. Shifting keeps you busy, and the idea is that once you have shifted you can have a new start and leave the old behind. So people keep shifting because with every move there is a lot to do and new things to learn and new friends to make and all that feels good for a little while. Until the feelings surface again and another shift is required. Sometimes it takes people a very long time to discover that they take their feelings with them wherever they go. It is impossible to move away from them. It can be necessary to shift location following a major loss, simply for financial or family reasons. But when this happens repeatedly, as in the case of one client who reported having shifted thirteen times in fourteen years following a significant family death, it is cause for concern and suggests a need to pause and evaluate what is happening.

Addictions

Getting inside your feelings can be avoided, denied, delayed or blocked by any number of means, but they all have the same purpose – to keep you from feeling. This can include medication. Although it has a place when trying to break the cycle of not eating, not sleeping, and continual fatigue, medication can be prolonged way beyond its usefulness. Many of the potions that are offered as a means to aid sleep or to make people feel better or less depressed also have the potential to be addictive.

At best, in my opinion, they only deal with the symptom and do not address the underlying cause of the sleeplessness or despondency. They certainly do not remove the loss, or the pain of grief that accompanies that loss. However medication suppresses it. And does so for as long as the medication is continued. Although I acknowledge that medication does have a place, my advice is to be wary of pills and alcohol. They provide only temporary relief from the pain and loneliness that is grief.

It is not just drugs and alcohol that are addictive. People can become addicted to processes as well. It is my belief that avoiding emotions lies at the root of many addictions. For example, the workaholic, the perfectionist, and the crisis-maker are all roles that can be addictive. I know these particular roles well because I discovered they were my own personal routes towards self-esteem and to avoid my own feelings. The point of an addiction is that it gives us a 'fix'; it makes us feel good. And as long as we have the addiction we don't have to worry about feeling awful, or about not having feelings (because at least we can keep busy and are useful). Retail therapy, gambling, sex, relationships, power, food, pain: any behaviour can be developed into an addiction, and the moment we need it to make us feel good (or to stop us feeling bad) then we are hooked. And we are still left with those distressing feelings that we haven't bothered to listen to or do anything about. They remain because the cause of our feelings has not been attended to. Maybe the event, or cause, happened so long ago that it has been forgotten. But the feelings remember, and listening to them will lead back to the cause.

Summary of Part II

When the process of getting inside your feelings is blocked, by whatever means, the result is that people experience depression. This depression is about pushing down inside yourself (or depressing) all of those feelings that want to come out. I pointed out earlier that sadness is often confused with depression and that disenfranchised grief is also frequently misinterpreted as depression. When depression manifests during grieving it is nearly always a symptom that leads to something else – commonly to blocked feelings. For some, the choice they make is to live with depression because it can be managed medically, and that seems preferable to undertaking this emotional work of grieving.

And so it is that people 'never really get over it'.

PART III

Making Adjustments and Learning How to Live Life Differently: How the Need for Change Can Be Blocked

Ordinarily this is where most people begin the work of grieving. They perhaps may not recognise it as such, but in order to continue living they make adjustments, little by little. If someone lives with chronic fatigue, they begin to learn what level of activity they can sustain without depleting their already reduced energy levels. When someone has broken a leg they learn to manoeuvre themselves on crutches. When a person emigrates from one culture to live in another, they adopt new forms of behaviour that ensure their acceptance. Although in principal these changes may seem obvious and to come about naturally, they can be complex and are not accomplished without effort. And our efforts can be, and often are, thwarted.

Comments that are flavoured with criticism, ridicule or teasing, or that suggest inadequacy, will be experienced as derogatory and hinder this part of the grieving process, because they increase the feeling of precariousness at a time when a person is already vulnerable. Other behaviours also block a person's progress with this task, but they are more difficult to recognise because of their subtlety and seductiveness. They are also condoned as acceptable social behaviour.

Dependency

The primary task of this part of grieving is to learn and develop skills that ensure independence. Should a person discover that independence is beyond their capabilities, then that in itself is another loss and cause for further grief which will need to be attended to.

Any adjustment or change to a previous way of life is difficult. It challenges our attitudes, beliefs and the adequacy of our current behaviour. It may mean that we have to retrain, learn new skills or rescind a decision that has already been implemented. And so we rail against this. We can argue that this is too difficult, takes too long, that we are too old or that we can't make decisions on our own. It is much easier to abdicate this responsibility, and to be comforted by others who are willing to assume this role.

In the early days of grief, people may see your limitations or difficulty and hasten to assist. And for an interim period, such assistance is legitimate and appreciated. Why is it then that such support so often goes awry and has the potential to lead to dependency? The dynamics usually involve one of two scenarios.

In the initial snowstorm of grief, the 'helper' rushes to assist in an endeavour to alleviate any 'upsetness' or perceived difficulty. At this point they feel useful and needed, and are pleased that they have been able to solve the problem. The grieving person however is usually left with conflicting feelings. On one hand they are grateful for this help. On the other, they are annoyed that they have been robbed of the opportunity to resolve the issue on their own and to make their own choices. Seldom is this ambivalence ever expressed. Rather people tend to remain silent and nurture the guilt that results from feeling annoyed because someone has been so good as to help them. And in the absence of any contrary feedback, the helper continues to assist long past the stage where it is warranted, in the mistaken belief that their input is what is wanted.

Alternatively, a grieving person may simply choose not to change. Again a 'helper' will undertake those chores the grief-stricken individual doesn't seem to be coping with. And the grieving person not only allows this to happen, but actively fosters its continuance. In fact they come to enjoy the 'help' and develop an expectation that not only will it continue, but that others will also see their need and render assistance. The 'helper' finds it difficult to withdraw, ultimately feels trapped by the circumstances they have unwittingly helped create, and then becomes resentful. Again, this resentment is seldom expressed directly. And in the absence of any contrary feedback, the grieving person continues to rely on the assistance and comes to expect it.

In both scenarios there is no honesty in the relationship, and neither have any clear boundaries or limits been set around the type or duration of assistance given or received. The result is that both parties ultimately feel trapped by these circumstances. In both scenarios the grieving person is not being helped to adjust and continue their independence. Their grieving has been effectively blocked and dependency created instead.

The best advice to any carer or 'helper' is for them to ask what is needed, and then to assist in a way that will enable the grieving person to solve their own dilemmas in a manner suitable for them. We particularly need to be aware of this when someone seeks to deal with a problem differently from the way we would.

A typical case is when an elderly, bereaved spouse faces living alone in the large family home with grounds that need to be maintained. I have learned that they are always very aware of their new circumstances and that changes will need to be made. However, the family can also recognise the problems to be faced, and unfortunately, make the decision that it is impractical for the solo parent to remain there. So they are shifted to smaller, more appropriate surroundings, or into a home. The family is relieved that the practical problems have been resolved, and return to their own home.

The recently bereaved spouse, who is already overwhelmed by grief, has now been forced to endure a further series of losses and to experience the subsequent emotional costs. At a time when they most needed the security provided by familiarity, the bereaved have to confront the loss of long time neighbours, community support, treasured possessions, independence, the understanding of family, and control of their own life (among other things). The grief that accompanies such major losses, and at a time of personal devastation, can cause major depression. It can be too much to bear. The adjustment that many elderly people then choose is to die.

What does help grieving is to provide the opportunity for people to adjust in their own time, and to explore some of their own solutions to problems. If it is at all possible, major decisions like shifting house are best deferred at least until the snowstorm phase of grief has settled. When a person is given time and supported in their grieving, problems and decisions will be faced as a matter of course, at a time and in a way that they can manage – provided the earlier traps that bring about dependency have been avoided. The solution may differ from the family's wishes, but the parent will be happier if things are resolved on their own terms. (Other options the parent could choose might be to pay for home help, or to barter their baking contribution at the church fête for a working bee on their grounds.)

Social Withdrawal

A state of dependency can be brought on just as readily by the bereaved or grieving person. They can for instance, accept myths as fact, and be unaware of what is required to resolve their grief. Or they may simply choose not to make any adjustment or develop new skills. And so at a time when they are overwhelmed by their loss and grief, they promote their own helplessness in order to elicit the assistance they so desperately require.

We all do this at times. Some of us learn to do it assertively. We are able to identify our need, and ask directly for this to be met, and in a way that all parties are agreeable to. Some people, however, have not developed this awareness, and rely instead on the game of 'Oh poor me'. This game is about manipulating others to look after them and some of the techniques that are utilised are blaming, complaining (as opposed to sharing), fear and guilt. They can also withdraw from life, work, friends or being involved socially in any way.

Such helplessness attracts well-meaning folk to look after these people, and their social contact is actually increased as a result. It also produces a 'nice' feeling of having been remembered and nurtured. This promotion of helplessness will continue for as long as there are people willing to fulfil their need. It is an effective strategy that blocks healthy grieving and, in fact, makes grieving seem unnecessary.

The most severe form of this withdrawal I have encountered involved a widow. Her husband had died ten years previously. A family member was concerned about her own inability to address her father's death and sought my assistance. She was perturbed that she alone had problems in this regard, and that her mother was coping well. On further inquiry I discovered just how her mother was coping. She had been on Valium since the day her husband had died, disposed of a flagon of sherry each evening, and had not ventured beyond the front gate since her spouse's death. I merely observed that she and I had a different definition of what it meant to be coping.

Another form of withdrawal not widely recognised is when people withdraw from themselves. The most common and socially acceptable form of this is to become totally devoted to looking after others. I must watch my words here, because caring for others is commendable, however, as in all things, there is a balance. And when someone is focused on avoiding their own issues and pain, any form of *caring for* another can become out of balance and turn into *care-taking*. Care-taking is when we make decisions, organise, and feel responsible for others, and it's a very effective means of withdrawing from oneself and negating one's own needs. Or, it can be care that is given in a distorted manner. Typical characteristics of this are self-neglect, assuming too much responsibility, inability to set boundaries, people-pleasing, controlling behaviour.

As I have mentioned earlier, there is a time when we all need to withdraw with our grief. And there is a time when such deliberate withdrawal no longer serves its purpose and actually becomes a deterrent to our grieving.

Summary to Part III

There is a realistic time-frame within which to make change after a loss. This will be different for each one of us as the changes required are directly related to the kind of loss we have experienced. Some adjustments are immediately obvious, while others emerge as we begin to live without what we have lost. Expecting people to make major decisions and further life changes during the initial time of upheaval is unrealistic, and can be detrimental to their well-being.

When a person steadfastly refuses to make any adjustment to accommodate their new circumstances they will not complete their grieving. Similarly, if they become dependent on the input of others to manage, the grieving process will also become blocked.

Any intervention that prevents a person from completing this aspect of grieving results in them simply not adjusting. They will strive to survive, and where there is no opportunity to adjust or support for them to do so, their focus will be on maintaining the status quo. This means they live in a form of denial, unable to function in the new reality.

I am reminded here of when my mother died. My father wished to remain in the family home and assumed that I (the only adult child who was single) would return home to take up where Mum had left off. Fortunately I had already learned how to say no, and explained that if he chose to live at home, he had to be able to do so independently. The initial negotiations were painful, for both of us, and although he later shifted, he did in fact continue to live on his own for a further twelve years. That would have been a very long time for both of us to have been caught in the dependency trap.

PART IV

The Spiritual Quest: How Establishing a Personal Philosophy and Re-engaging With Life Can Be Blocked

We all have a tendency to defer consideration of these weighty matters until directly confronted with them. But grief is the inevitable consequence of loving and will come to us all. It is during these times of personal challenge that we seek to find meaning and purpose for without a life philosophy, the alternative is despair. And so grieving and growth in our spiritual dimensions are inextricably wound together. Fear is the single, biggest factor that blocks the task of grieving and of successfully embracing life again.

Fear

Anyone working through the grieving process will have discovered that it is painful, and that this pain comes as the result of having loved. There is consequently a very real fear of being hurt in the same way, and to the same extent, again. People therefore instinctively, almost unconsciously, do things that will protect themselves from being hurt. Unfortunately the things they do to avoid future pain are the same things that prevent them from becoming involved. Fear becomes an impediment to intimacy.

Fear can also accompany the efforts of those who begin to re-establish themselves. There is fear of the unknown, fear of being on your own, fear of what other people will think, fear that you won't make it. And for those who are bereaved, there is the fear of being disloyal to the deceased. This is usually quick to surface when people discover they are enjoying themselves, and it definitely becomes an issue as they merge back into life and find themselves becoming attracted to someone else.

In our death-denying death-defying culture, people experience a very real fear when confronting their own mortality. There is little in the responses of others to assist them. 'What are you thinking about that for, for heaven's sake' or 'Do you have to be so morbid?' or 'Why worry about that when you've plenty of living to do?' are normal rebuttals to any serious exploration of thanatology. Yet when we have experienced a personal crisis or been in close proximity to death, our awareness is changed and we can no longer ignore the finiteness of humanity.

From this point there is a yearning for insight into the meaning and purpose of life in general, and our own life in particular. There is a growing consciousness of our reasons for being here.

And questions about suffering, life after death, and is there a God all need answers. Active searching, reading, and debate are necessary to address these issues, as is the freedom to engage in this exploration. Yet again, fear may restrict people. Fear of imagined consequences, fear of eternal damnation, and fear of rejection are ways people become inhibited.

So fear can make prisoners of us all – and if it does, grieving is never completed. The outcome is to live life at a superficial level that does not demand involvement. The tragedy is that the individual is neither able to give, or receive, love.

All too frequently people begin to build protective walls around themselves. Walls of denial, or indifference or silence; they can be walls built from rationalising or from creating a myriad of rules to control other people's behaviour. Walls can be constructed from perfectionism or from having an excessive concern for others. When we withdraw from anything or anyone we build a wall. Even humour and sex can be fostered to wall status as they close off intimacy. Just about anything can be used to wall us off from ourselves, our fears, the real issue, our grief, or another person.

Walls may have a plastic coated 'niceness' or be covered in barbed wire. But walls have several purposes. They create the illusion of safety and they keep other people from coming too close and touching us on a sore spot. They do not afford protection from any fears that you are seeking to escape. They also prevent you from loving, and from being loved in return. And they hinder grieving and healing.

Chapter Summary

I hope that highlighting these behaviours has provided some insight into why people 'never really get over it'. Any intervention that restricts a person from undertaking, or completing, any one of these areas of grieving, means that their grief will not be resolved. It will simply settle like the snowstorm, and be reactivated at any time with the slightest shake or reminder.

It is my opinion that we have not been well equipped to understand and deal with grief. A lack of education, misinformation and stereotypical expectations all contrive to prevent us from developing healthy social norms with which to express it. Consequently there are many social inhibitors that keep people stuck in the grief. And because our learning has been not to express grief, it is true that many 'never really get over it'.

Grief however, is common to the whole of human kind. And how we learn to express that grief is culturally learned. Other cultures deal with grief differently. Each has its own rituals, beliefs and social norms that allow for grief to be given expression. This can be the basis for more difficulty. When a person is inducted into one way of expressing grief, it becomes restrictive when they live in another culture. Our culture has not yet learned to fully appreciate differences, let alone tolerate them. And so it is that in many instances the grieving practices of those from another culture are often labelled as wrong, offensive, or stupid. Each culture has developed burial rites and grieving behaviour. All are different. Each is legitimate. But there is little in our culture that affords recognition or acceptance of this. And the silence or suppression with which the majority (in New Zealand Pakeha culture) responds to grief is not a healthy alternative which people from other cultures wish to adopt. Both our culture and religious beliefs influence our attitudes and emotional expression and when there is an impediment to either, grieving can't be resolved. This is another reason why many people 'never really get over it'.

Grieving for losses of long ago is also difficult. It means going back and working through pain that has been avoided for years. It is particularly arduous because people do not understand why someone is grieving when there is currently no apparent cause. When told that a person is grieving for the loss of their childhood, innocence or creativity as the result of being sexually abused during childhood, people are often unable or unwilling to understand. They respond naively by suggesting that the past is best left in the past or to let bygones be bygones. The social supports that may have been available when the loss occurred are all too frequently absent when these losses are honoured and grieved as adults. When grieving is separated from the loss and expressed at a different time, it is a more complex and difficult experience. This lack of understanding and support is another root cause for why many more people 'never really get over it'.

Another factor that can inhibit grieving is a clash or conflict of social and professional roles. I share my own experience to illustrate this. I was working as a funeral director at the time my mother died, and some members of my family had the expectation that I would attend to all the necessary arrangements. My boss, however, clearly and firmly informed everyone that in this instance I was not the funeral director. I was the daughter, and needed to grieve as such. In that moment I was immediately relieved of professional responsibility, any possible burden, and the potential of conflict within the family.

I was simply able to grieve for my mum.

Often the doctor, nurse, minister, lawyer or therapist are regularly expected to deliver their expertise freely while their more immediate family role and needs are overlooked. However, it can be satisfying to operate from the professional role and receive the gratification of others. It can also be a marvellous way of avoiding the discomfort of grief. And yet again, it can result in many people not 'really getting over it'.

Although each area of grieving has been mentioned in sequence, work can be undertaken in each area simultaneously or in any order. There is, however, a natural order and continuity to the process. It is only in facing the new reality that we perceive a need to adjust our behaviour. And in allowing ourselves to experience the hurt that accompanies such loss and change, we question why and seek understanding beyond what the intellect has to offer and explore the realms of the metaphysical.

Most commonly grieving begins when people focus on adjusting their behaviour in order to survive and accommodate the loss they have experienced. Unfortunately, having done that, the majority believe that their grieving is complete. And so the process is never completed. The work of the emotional and spiritual dimensions is not attended to.

Grieving can be interrupted or halted by any one of the interventions described in this chapter, or any combination of them. These interventions can be caused by the actions of others, or they can be self-inflicted. They are the key reasons why people never really get over their grief.

Food for Thought

This is an exercise designed to illustrate how the responses shown below interfere with grieving and why they are unhelpful.

The work of grieving involves:

I. Coming to believe what has happened and accepting that reality

II. Getting inside your feelings

III. Making changes and learning how to live life differently

IV. A spiritual quest

Common Responses

a) Not mentioning the loss or death

b) Avoiding references to the deceased by name

c) Trying to avoid saying anything that might 'upset' the other person

d) Telling the grieving what they should do

e) Taking on responsibility for the grieving person, and their problems, and then feeling trapped

f) Indicating grieving has a time-frame (e.g. you should be over that by now)

g) Giving false reassurances

h) Using cliches in your responses

i) Telling them of someone else you knew who has had a similar experience

j) Trying to find a positive thought or aspect for your response

k) Making a decision for the bereaved without checking it out with them
l) Forcing the grieving person to socialise
m) Telling someone they shouldn't feel guilty and then using logical argument to explain why
n) Showing or communicating surprise or disapproval over what the grieving person is doing, or intends to do
o) Mentioning my beliefs about death, God, and what happens in the hereafter without being asked, or tried to convince the other person they were wrong in their beliefs

Consider each response and think which of the four areas of work it would prevent the grieving person completing. For example, responses a) and b) obstruct all four areas of recovery. It is hard to face and accept reality when you cannot talk about it; silence avoids any display of feelings; it gives no assistance in the adjustment process; and it creates difficulties in re-establishing a social environment.

Personal Exercise

Is your grieving fully resolved?

If you have encountered, or engaged in, any of the responses referred to throughout this chapter, it may be that your ability to grieve has been affected. Here are some questions that are offered as a guideline for checking how complete the process is for you.

- Are you unable to talk about your loss?
- Do you experience great emotional pain or despair when you do talk about it?
- Do you prevent yourself from becoming attached to anything again?
- Are you afraid to love again?
- Have you become socially withdrawn because of your experience?
- Do you still use present tense when you refer to your loss?
- Are your dreams or thoughts unpleasant or disturbing?
- Have you become irrationally overprotective with others as a result?
- Do you find yourself resenting other people's happiness or well-being and then being spiteful toward them because of it?
- Have you developed an ongoing health problem since the loss occurred?
- Do you still avoid anything or anyone that brings back memories?

- Is your eating or drinking excessive, or different from your regular pattern?

If you answer yes to any of these questions it may be that your grieving is not complete.

If you answered yes three or more times, I suggest you seek support to identify and then move beyond any possible blockage.

Summary of Key Points

The Work of Grieving	How This Gets Blocked
I. Coming to believe what has happened and accepting reality.	Comparing losses and grief. Reducing, altering or denying either the facts, significance or irreversibility of the loss. (Known as minimising the event)
II. Getting inside your feelings.	Avoiding feelings. Learning not to feel. Shifting and keeping busy. Rationalising. Addictive behaviours.
III. Making changes and learning how to live life differently.	Not developing new skills. Becoming dependent on others. Permanent social withdrawal.
IV. A spiriual quest.	Fear of being hurt again. Fear of own mortality.

Social Inhibitors	Outcome for Grieving Person
Some losses and grief are considered to be socially unacceptable and are therefore negated.	Denial.
Social roles and conditioning that we adopt. The family system and how it deals with grief.	Depression.
Culture and religious beliefs influence emotional expression and attitudes about what is appropriate and acceptable grieving.	Not able to adapt, or adjust to new situation.
Diminished or non-existent social networks.	Not able to give or receive love.

8 *Myth: I should be able to do this on my own.*

> *Reality: Grieving is a social process. It cannot be completed in isolation.*

This is arguably the greatest paradox of grief. At a time when you are most affected by grief you will seek privacy. However, we need people to help us with our grieving.

Historically, in Western, Pakeha culture, grief has not been associated with general loss, and because of this people denied its impact and struggled in private. This conspiracy of silence has been a fertile breeding ground for many of our current attitudes. It was, however, permissible to grieve following a death. Traditionally there were a number of communal ceremonies following the death, and the bereaved were distinguished by a change in physical appearance. They wore clothes of different colours that depicted the passage of their mourning. Shaving, or the lack of it, conveyed a similar message. There was a formal withdrawal from society followed by a period of seclusion. And at the end of a designated period of mourning (which depended on one's relationship to the deceased), a formal, but gradual, re-entry into society was organised. Death and mourning have always been socially recognised. Loss and grieving, on the other hand, have not.

Nowadays we have no such established mourning customs and the fact that grieving is a natural and inevitable consequence of major loss is still not widely recognised. We therefore fail to provide the ongoing support or comfort people require. Instead, in many instances, we avoid their anguish and leave them to 'get over it' on their own. In the absence of social messages to the contrary, grieving people have assumed it is their sole responsibility to recover from the impact of personal tragedy. This can mean that they are left in an isolated position. Isolation kills. We now know from studies of orphaned children and animals that babies wither away if they aren't held and cuddled frequently. The clinical term for this is 'failure to thrive'. Even as adults, without support systems we too fail to thrive. We all need to be heard, to be valued and to be guided. No one can heal this pain but you, and it's almost impossible to heal it by yourself.

As mentioned previously, there will be times when it is necessary for you to seek the consolation of your own company and to retreat from others. This will be especially so during the intense snowstorm of grief. But if you are to heal from your experience of loss, then it is essential that you involve other people.

When to involve others raises difficulties because we have none of the previously prescribed social customs which signal our readiness to others. As a consequence those who have not had a similar experience are unable to comprehend the enormity or intensity of your grief, and will frequently pressure you to socialise long before you are ready. You must retain control over this for yourself, and your feelings will be your best guide. Honour them at all times. To agree to an outing when it is the last thing you feel like doing is dishonest and will cause you more grief. What you will lose is respect for your own needs and control over your own recovery. However in not accepting the invitation there is always risk involved because you may jeopardise a friendship. Therefore when choosing to decline a social invitation, always give a genuine explanation and encourage people to continue to ask you, because there will be a day when you are ready. Mistakenly, people will make a polite deferral and blame it on other factors.

The professional roles of many people engenders them to be more comfortable with supporting others than accepting support; as a result they can be reluctant to declare their need and have others become involved. But the expectation that you should be able to complete this process entirely on your own is unrealistic and unnecessarily punitive. To a greater or lesser degree, we need other people to assist with our grieving in each stage of the process.

Four Social Tasks
Facing Reality
The most basic and helpful thing anyone can do to help this phase is to talk. We need to tell our story over and over, because talking helps us to hear what we are thinking, and this brings insight. We need people to listen to us. Having someone who will listen (as opposed to giving advice or trying to fix the

problem) validates us and our experience. All too frequently people think that their painful reactions to an event are abnormal, and that they too are abnormal because they cannot control those reactions. Talking and being listened to helps us to integrate what has happened and come to realise that our responses are normal, and that the event is (to us) abnormal.

There are many activities that will assist people to face reality. They may, for example, need to visit places, talk to witnesses, search medical or police records or attend judicial processes. To have the company and comfort of a support person during these times is invaluable. Throughout this course of action good friends will encourage honesty and challenge any playing down of the event. We need people who can afford us respect, so that we can come to respect our grief and grieving.

Expressing feelings

Most of us find it embarrassing to let our feelings show. But for those who are committed to their own recovery, it is imperative to express emotion. It helps to have selected people with whom to do this. We need people around us whom we can trust, and who will be non-judgemental. We need to be comforted during times of distress, even if that amounts simply to a gentle word or a passing of the tissues.

After the times when we have felt most exposed, we need to know that people are still accepting of us, despite the feelings we have displayed. Our pain is the result of our attachment, and we need people to give testimony to both our loving and our loss, so that we can accept our feelings. By honouring our own feelings we are honouring ourselves: it is also the first step towards understanding and respecting the feelings of another.

Feeling Supported

As we are faced with making a myriad of lifestyle adjustments, we need practical assistance from people with expertise and skills. And for them to offer assistance without any suggestion of inadequacy on our part.

As we regain our independence, we need to explore our ideas with other people. Having your own personal team of cheerleaders for ongoing encouragement is a wonderful support. Overall, we need people who can be dignified in their response to us so that we can move beyond disparaging our own shortcomings, and reorganise our lives with dignity.

Re-establishment

At this point, when the snowstorm has settled and healing has begun, people begin to socialise again, to whatever degree they feel comfortable with.

We simply cannot be sociable on our own. We need other people with whom to enjoy our social pursuits and who will be patient with our tentativeness and limited periods of endurance. When the days are long, and we are in a bad space, it is helpful to have contact with others who have weathered a similar experience. From their presence and sharing we come to realise that recovery is possible, and their knowledge is expressed in a way that demands nothing from us. They understand the need to explore all matters spiritual and are open to having their own beliefs scrutinised. These people become our inspiration. And it is through such people who give us their patience and generosity of spirit that we learn to love again.

Grief in the workplace

Whether we care to admit it or not, when we are grieving, those around us are always affected by it. There are those who still believe that they can divorce themselves from what is happening in their personal life when they go to work. It is their way of coping, but such thinking is simplistic. If we leave 'the personal' part of ourselves at home, we have already reduced our capacity to think and feel, and restricted our working potential. Those around us notice the changes in our demeanour and the way we interact with them.

Research has identified that when people return to work after bereavement leave or following an absence because of personal tragedy, the accident rate increases. This is because people who are tired, unable to concentrate, and preoccupied with a life changing event, return to work where they are expected to make responsible decisions and operate complex technical equipment and machinery. Given their state of mind and depleted physical resources, accidents are a natural consequence.

Accidents are not inevitable, however. When a person is willing to acknowledge their grief and current state of wellbeing, employers and colleagues can be kept informed, and involved. I have worked with a few enlightened organisations that have been willing to accommodate changes to assist their staff. Buddy programmes have been established, system checks put in place, further time out made available, counselling services provided, glide time introduced for the person concerned, work tasks redistributed and a less demanding work focus organised temporarily. When the approach is co-operative, there is no end to the creative solutions that can be produced. Without exception I have discovered that when the experience of a grieving employee is made overt and they are assisted in this way, their recovery is quicker and there is less disruption in the workplace.

Unfortunately such a co-operative approach is not the norm. I have found it more common for employees to be fearful of their employers discovering their diminished working capacity, and to fear that they will be punished because of it. The majority of employers on the other hand, appear to be ill-informed about grief and its effects and so have unrealistic expectations of their employees during this time. So rather than engaging in grief education for all concerned, the employee plays 'I'm fine', and the employer demands 'You'd better be'. And accidents can happen. Sometimes they are fatal.

Directly or indirectly, consciously or unconsciously, others are affected when we grieve. To deny this fact is selfish. It is selfish because it denies someone else their experience, and the opportunity for them to deal with it. It prevents communication and feedback about our own progress. I well remember when my boss approached me about six months on from my mother's death. Firmly but gently, he described aspects of my working behaviour which suggested to him that I was angry. 'Deal with it' was the message, 'or you will not continue to deal directly with the clients.' I was mortified. I was also very angry, at my boss. I was angry that he thought I was angry about my mother's death (when I didn't consider I was) and that he had the gall to tell me so. I experienced a range of emotions, but ultimately it was my passion for my work that took me to counselling. It took a while, but guess what? I discovered I was angry. The root cause was not immediately obvious but eventually I uncovered it. My father's behaviour had been the cause of much terror for me when I was a child, and as long as I could remember he had always had health problems. As a result, my expectation had been that he would predecease my mother. In fact it occurred the other way round. And indeed, I was furious. However, this unidentified hostility was obvious to all but me. It is thanks to my boss and his feedback that I was able to progress in my grieving.

Just because we may not be aware of some aspect of our behaviour doesn't mean that it isn't happening. Unfortunately this is the source of a lot of unpleasantness in the workplace as concealed feelings are dealt with indirectly and displaced onto colleagues or 'difficult' customers. It behoves a willingness on our part to actively monitor and attend to our own grieving process. This can be assisted by being open to assistance.

Support Groups

It always amuses me that the people who speak most vociferously against support groups and counselling, are those who have no experience of either. Admittedly in participating in a group we need to beware those with rigid and constrictive philosophies. But a support group is precisely that – support. It will offer grief education, information about related services, the support of a network of people who are coping with similar circumstances, and help to develop your recovery.

In the bereavement support groups I am involved with, small groups (six to ten people) meet one night a week for six weeks. Each night has a topic that structures my input and group discussion. Apart from becoming better informed about their own situation, several things occur during the course. First of all, people find it an enormous relief to discover that what they are experiencing is normal and that everyone else can relate to what they describe. Until this discovery, each has secretly harboured the fear that they might be going mad. Second, they encounter empathy, rather than sympathy, and so learn to modify their responses to each other and, by implication, to others outside the group. Finally they begin to develop effective strategies that help give expression to their grief, and assist with their response to the demands of others.

Group members invariably express surprise when they find they enjoy coming to the group. It is, they say, the one place where they can be honest and be accepted without judgement. They discover the benefits of being able to talk freely about their circumstances, and express relief at dispelling the myths that have controlled their social behaviour.

An invitation to our support group is offered approximately six months following the bereavement. It is generally about this time that the effects of the snowstorm are first beginning to abate, and when many incorrectly interpret this as the end of their grief. Our invitation is also timed to coincide with the period when initial supports are diminishing and the social expectation that 'You should be over it by now' is beginning to emerge. Support is often necessary to endure a process that lasts a lot longer than society is prepared to tolerate. We now accommodate a growing number of people who ask to attend the group many years on from a death.

Admittedly, joining a support group must always be a personal choice. But don't knock it before you have explored what it has to offer. 'I don't need it' is a common refrain. I wonder on what criteria people have made their self-assessment, and marvel that an opportunity for growth and healing is equated with weakness or 'neediness': needs are basic human attributes.

An alternative to a group experience is working one on one. Again the idea of attending counselling or therapy may still meet with derision in our culture, so that many do not acknowledge that they are recieving help through counselling. However, counselling can be helpful when we have few friends or are lacking social support. More often than not it is necessary when grief is delayed, and does not accompany the loss. It is essential when the grieving process becomes hindered and results in pathological mourning. Counselling is not a place where crazy people go, but rather where sane people go for help when everything around them has gone crazy. Nowhere is that more applicable than when we need to grieve. It also indicates acceptance of responsibility for one's health and well-being. With no formal education about grief or the grieving process, where else are we to learn?

Summary

I hope these few points illustrate why we cannot resolve grief on our own. To steadfastly refuse help is selfish and denies the negative effect we may have on others. Coping does not mean that you have to manage on your own. I do not understand why stoicism is still sanctified.

Food For Thought

A Blessing for Your Journey

May the road always rise to meet you
May the wind be always at your back
May the sun shine warm upon your face
May the rain fall soft on your back
And until we meet again
May the Good Lord hold you soft in
the hollow of His hand.

Celtic blessing

Personal Reflection

We live with a number of rooms inside us. Different topics are discussed in each of these rooms. The best room is always open to a wide range of family and friends. Another room is more private and reserved for those closest to us. There is another room where we allow no-one in, not even our partners or children, for it is a room of the most intimate thoughts we keep safe. There is one more room that is kept locked, and we don't even enter it ourselves. Here we keep hidden all the mysteries we can not solve and all the pain and sorrows we wish to forget.

Consider the events in your life that have resulted in loss and grief. Then visit each room and see which event you keep there, and to whom you can talk to about these things.

Topics for a wide range of family and friends	My private room
Topics for those closest to us	My locked room

Summary of Key Points

- Grieving is a social process.

- A lack of established social customs means that grieving people are not provided with the ongoing support and comfort they require.

- Throughout grieving, we need people around us by whom we can feel accepted, listened to, loved and supported.

- When employers are advised, changes can be made in the workplace and accidents prevented.

- Other people have valuable feedback to give us about our grieving behaviour and our progress.

- Support groups can be helpful. There is much to be gained by learning from others who have had a similar experience.

- Counselling is where sane people go for help when they realise that everything around them has gone crazy.

- Coping does not mean that you have to manage on your own.

9 Myth: *I must not wallow in self-pity.*

> **Reality:** *Allowing yourself to grieve is caring for yourself. It is not self-pity.*

Self-care is something that many are unfamiliar with. It is not a concept that is usually promoted in our society, and any behaviour directed towards meeting our own needs can be labelled as selfish. Admittedly this is a complex subject about which others have written more extensively than I can here. Suffice to say that in our society people are generally more accepting, and in need of, relationships which foster and ensure mutual dependency and care. As a consequence, when we tend to our own needs, others feel rejected. Any effort to be independent can be perceived as threatening, and lead to accusations of selfishness. Which works. Such accusations engender guilt and as a result we fall into self-doubt and halt self-care.

The implied bargain in any such dependent relationship is that 'You be there to look after me, and I'll be there to look after you'. And while you tend diligently to their needs, in the midst of your grief you discover that in fact they are not looking after you – that was a fantasy. Only you can do your grieving. Only you know what you need. Only you can meet your needs. Others can help us with their support and compassion, but only you can heal your hurt. The alternative is to live the fantasy and expect another to look after you, and to be forever frustrated as their efforts fall short of your expectations and requirements.

There is no longer guidance from social rituals showing us how to react to grief. As a consequence, you will often be left alone during the period when you most need help and comfort. Any expectations you may have that society will understand your needs and take care of you, are unrealistic. You will discover however, that you become socially acceptable again if you act as though nothing of substance has happened. And so we come to chastise ourselves when we feel sorry for ourselves and want to look after ourselves. How absurd! Who else is going to do it?

Self-care is being a loving and tolerant friend to yourself. Self-care is about attending to our own development so that we grow to maturity in all aspects of our personality. If we can achieve this, then we can share our completeness with other people, rather than demand that they meet our needs and thus make us complete. Self-care is recognising who and what we are. Self-care is the ability to nurture ourselves, and to do so before we give out to others. Self-care is being self-centred.

No doubt these words will cause some controversy, because we have been educated to believe that self-centred means self-ish. But if we are not centred in ourselves, then we are centred on something or someone else. And how can we know who we are if we have no centre to our being? The way the majority of people solve this dilemma is to comply with other's expectations, whether these are right for them or not. They therefore define themselves according to their fantasies of what other people want of them.

Self-care is legitimate. It means loving ourselves and not betraying ourselves, and this comes from living in accordance with our own truth, however we have defined this. When we are in touch with who we are, we are in touch with a greater force and can allow our spirit full expression. To deny this, or ignore our own needs, is a sign of spiritual depletion. Self-care is therefore necessary for our spiritual growth.

Self-pity, on the other hand, is when we think of ourselves as contemptible. Someone is full of self-pity when they despise themselves, or the fact that they have needs. People are also full of self-pity when they carry regrets, and when they refuse to allow others to help or contribute to their well-being. Those who live in the role of victim and avoid personal responsibility are living in self-pity. Self-pity and selfish hold hands.

However, grieving is a natural, normal process. It is our response when we experience a loss of any kind. It is the means by which we heal from the hurt involved when detaching ourselves from what we have loved. It is painful, takes time to work through, and requires effort on our part. But grieving is not self-pity. Rather we are caring for ourselves.

Let me put it another way. Here is my earlier description of the snowstorm of grief in pictorial form:

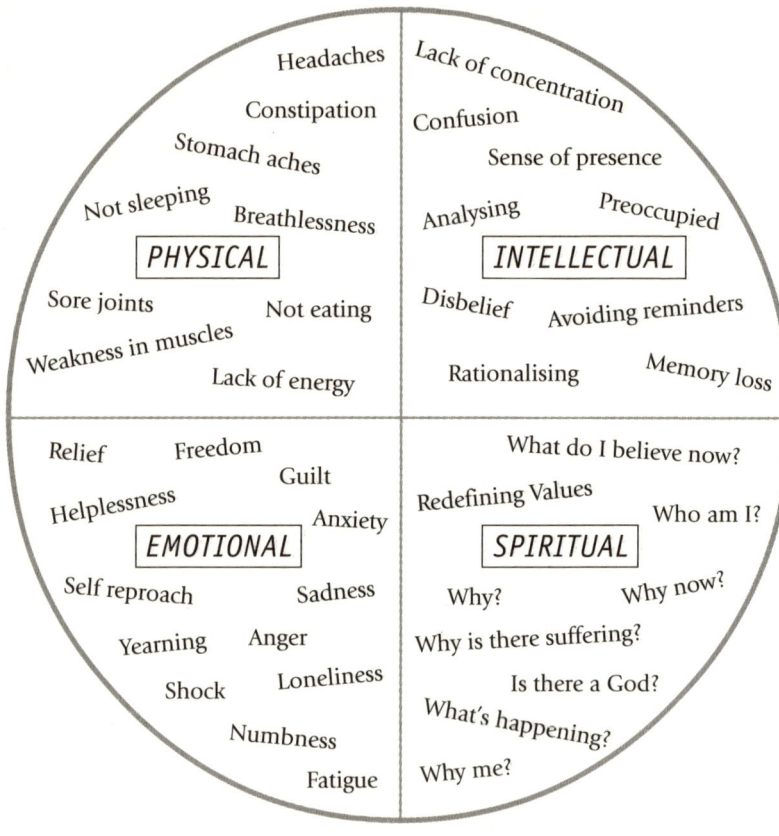

If this were a friend standing in the midst of such over-whelming grief, would you feel compassion for them? Would you want to help? How would you respond? I have a notion that your heart would go out to them and that you would at least stand by them, maybe even love them all the more.

Now imagine it is you standing in the midst of this picture, and allow yourself to feel some compassion for yourself. You are allowed to feel sorry for yourself. We are all allowed to feel sorry for ourselves when we are in the midst of such circumstances. Rather than make things even more difficult, learn to be gentle with yourself, and allow yourself to experience the same feelings you would have for a friend. Be your own best friend.

For most of us, grief is one of the most painful experiences of our life. We struggle to make sense of it and to find reasons for our loss. I have used the image of a snowstorm in an attempt to put grief into perspective and so make it more manageable. There are many aspects of the snowstorm that illustrate why self-care is so important.

- A snowstorm is disorienting. White-out conditions prevail, and all sense of direction is quickly lost. Communication systems often break down and long-range vision becomes restricted.

- We have no control over when or where a snowstorm occurs, and the duration of each varies considerably. At times they can be most unseasonable and defy even geographic location.

- Travelling in a snowstorm can be dangerous and extra care and attention is required.

- Staying out in a snowstorm for any period of time is exhausting.

- It takes time for a snowstorm to blow itself out.

Similarly, in the midst of grief people become muddled, feel they have no control over what is happening, and are continually tired. Extra care and attention is required in order to endure it. At some point, we will be faced with the dilemma of choosing whether the snowstorm will become an endpoint or a journey. When it becomes an endpoint, self-pity emerges. When we choose to journey on, self-care is imperative.

Here then are some suggestions for a self-care plan.

- Try and maintain your regular routines. This may be easier said than done, but make the effort to eat and ensure you get enough rest. Prepare food you enjoy, and eat when you are hungry. Similarly, sleep when you are tired, and ensure that you at least rest even if you are unable to sleep. Try to maintain your regular household or daily routines: e.g. shop, clean, do other chores as usual, to give yourself stability in the chaos of change.

- Regular exercise is also important, even if it is less strenuous than you are used to. Go for a walk in the evening. It is easy to stop exercising when feeling tired, but even a gentle walk will take you out of the house and afford some time that is free from all other demands.

- Take one day at a time and have a plan for each day. Include one task and some time for yourself each day. This will provide a structure and will also ensure that everything is attended to. Learn to be flexible because your needs may change from day to day.

- Keep in touch with friends. If you cannot muster the energy to go visiting, make a brief phone call on a regular basis. Allow new people to enter your life, because it can be a relief to spend time with someone who is not aware of your loss and that you are grieving.

- Schedule a treat for yourself every week. Be creative, but remember the aim is to be nice to yourself. Eat out, have a massage, walk on the beach, take the phone off the hook and soak in a bath. Make a list of things you enjoy doing, choose one each week and carry it out. This is a wonderful gift to give yourself.

- Fight loneliness and cry when you want to. The small hours of the night are when this most often happens and personally I think there is nothing like a teddy bear to help. My teddy, Barnaby, is always there when I need to talk or cry, no matter what time of the day or night. You can cuddle a soft toy till the fur rubs off and they don't complain. They are excellent listeners and never interrupt. Barnaby has never told me what I 'should' do, or offered unwanted advice. He has never broken a confidence. And he has never been critical of my language or how I speak. His loyalty and devotion to me is a real comfort. I have a notion that pets may fill this role for some, but my cat is not too fond of cuddles, so Barnaby it is.

- Stay in control of your own life. There are many who want to rescue people in snowstorms. And initially that can be a welcome respite. But having rescued you, there are those who believe they then have the right to make decisions for you and tell you what to do. And all the while the snowstorm continues. Avoid making hasty decisions about major issues and learn to say no. Developing assertiveness skills will be invaluable, and will also help teach you about personal boundaries and how to implement them.

- Be aware of what expectations you have for yourself. Different energy levels, tiredness and a diminished concentration span may mean that your expectations need to be modified for a time. Have a realistic time-frame within which to expect recovery; it will last longer than a few months. Periodically look back on your own progress and take notice of small improvements.

- Plan ahead for anniversaries and holiday times. Many people wait in dread as the anniversary of the death or loss approaches, or for Christmas to come and go. Be proactive. Decide what you want to do, rather than what friends or relatives expect you to, or what will make them more comfortable. Your life has changed, so to continue as if nothing has happened helps no-one, least of all you. Inform others of your changed needs and be specific about your preferences. These critical times will also place additional demands on your time and emotions, so be aware of your limitations.

- Build a support system for yourself and use it often. When people want to do things for you, let them. Be open to the idea of involving others, including professionals. It may be that this most recent loss has triggered other memories and unresolved grief, and guidance in how to deal with this may be necessary.

Being deliberate about your self-care may be hard, and it may be helpful to enlist the support of a friend, employer or partner in order to carry it out. But allow yourself breathing space and expect changes in your moods and perspective. Grieving is like working overtime. Not only is life more complicated, but all energy is siphoned into mental and emotional resolution. Grieving is nature's way of healing the mind and heart from the greatest injury of all. Allow yourself the privilege of limping till your wounds have healed and you can learn to run again. The metaphor of the snowstorm is also realistic. Those who continue to walk in a snowstorm invariably get lost or suffer from exhaustion. Sometimes the wisest thing is to ride the storm and wait until it abates rather than to continue the journey amidst its fury.

Allowing yourself this breathing space is related to nurturing yourself. It's about doing nice things for yourself that you would suggest to someone else. And when we care for ourselves in this way we feel valued, loved and in touch with who we really are. Wallowing in self-pity means struggling on, despite all that is happening, and waiting forever until someone comes along to love you, fix your life, and make you feel good. Some people who wallow and wait never recover.

Another concept that is seldom linked with self-care is forgiveness. Forgiveness nearly always implies our behaviour towards others, yet sometimes we can be very harsh on ourselves, particularly following tragedy. We are apt to hold ourselves accountable, believing that something we did, or didn't do, contributed to the event. This may or may not be so, but ultimately such thinking influences the way we treat ourselves. To be forgiving of yourself is also to be a friend to yourself, and is a necessary step toward healing.

What exactly does it mean to forgive? This is something I have struggled long and hard to understand. No-one has ever been able to explain to me what it actually means and how to do it. Here are some of my current thoughts on forgiving.

Forgiving does not mean forgetting. That is impossible, because whatever has caused me grief is a part of my experience and contributes to who I am. When something of importance has occurred in our lives it is usually impossible to simply forget it. Even if we shut out the memory, our being (or spirit) will still carry the knowledge of what has happened.

Forgiving does not mean overlooking, justifying or excusing the abuse or transgressions of another. Neither does it mean denying your own experiences and the pain, hurt and anger that results from them. And it is definitely not about saying it's okay to continue the abusive action. Neither person benefits from any of these strategies, although it does allow the disrespectful or careless behaviour to continue. Even an abuser is abused when we allow harmful behaviour to continue.

I have come to think that forgiveness is precisely that. What have I got 'for giving' to someone (or myself), right here, right now? When I consider this in regard to one of my abusers, I used to think the answer was nothing. In truth what I had 'for giving' to him was hate, resentment, hurt and a wanting to kill him, or at least a wishing to see him suffer in a similar way. Now, having worked through my grieving with the help of several professionals, what I have 'for giving' to him is some understanding of who he was and why he acted as he did, some compassion, and a wish for him to experience some healing from his injuries as I have. I am now able to visualise him surrounded by soft coloured light, or wrapping him in a rainbow or sending him flowers. And I feel the better now 'for giving' him these different things.

At this stage in my life, I also have benefited 'for giving' to myself. Once all I ever gave myself was a hard time. I had end-less supplies of guilt and shame and a need to be punished for what had happened to me (because I assumed it was my re-sponsibility). Now I give myself some love and acceptance. I allow myself to have fun and play. I can be who I am, in any situation without need to apologise, and I allow myself to continually dream a greater vision of who I want to be. I am working on giving myself permission to fully express all of my creative ability. I believe I have gone a long way to forgiving myself. I'm certainly a lot happier as a result.

Forgiving is remembering and facing the reality of what-ever has happened. It is working through all the horror and pain and multiple feelings that accompany this reality. And then it is about being able to accept what is, and let it be. We cannot forget our past; it is part of what makes us who we are, and it is the source of our understanding, compassion and empathy. When we have left our baggage behind and can ex-tend these attributes to another without the need to tell our own story, we are forgiving.

Forgiving is more than words. It is behaviour that clothes an attitude. Forgiveness is not an event, but an ongoing process.

And to give to yourself is not wallowing in self-pity.

Personal Reflection

A self-care plan

Divide the pie into quarters and list those things you do (or could do) to look after yourself physically, intellectually, emotionally and spiritually.

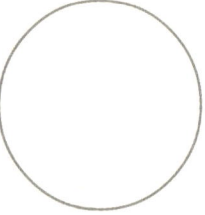

Now consider how much of your time you devote to each area of your life, and how you could incorporate these activities. Some suggested headings are listed below. Divide the first pie up according to how it is now. On the second pie, rearrange the size of the sections according to how you would like it to be.

Home	Partner	Myself
Work	Children	My health
Leisure	Friends	Personal growth
Community	Family	Spiritual needs

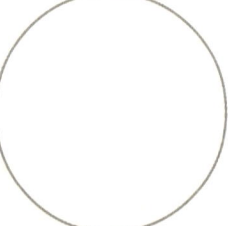

How it is now   *How I would like it to be*

Food For Thought

It's Never to Late to Have a Happy Childhood

You are very special
You may never had the opportunity
   to believe in your specialness
You may believe it today.

Claudia Black

Summary of Key Points

- Self-care is different from self-pity.

- Only you know your needs and can meet them. Only you
  can heal your heart.

- Self-care is being a loving and tolerant friend to yourself.

- It is important to have a self-care plan and to practise it.

- When we care for ourselves we feel valued, loved and in
  touch with who we really are.

- Forgiveness is a necessary part of healing and self-care.

- When we allow ourselves to grieve, we are not wallowing
  in self-pity.

10 *Myth: Best leave them alone to get over it.*

Reality: People cannot get over loss on their own. They need to maintain their connection with you, and yes, you can help.

At first glance the above sentiment seems reasonable. It appears to convey a thoughtfulness that is most concerned with the needs of the grieving person. When we look deeper we find that the underlying (perhaps unconscious) motive behind this expression may be to avoid our own discomfort. You may want to avoid becoming involved, or you may feel awkward about not knowing how to respond. Either way, using this myth lets you off the hook and from having to look too closely at your own reactions. But being left alone by people who were considered to be friends adds hurt to an already painful experience.

This aloneness is like a void for which there is no explanation and the grieving person is left to interpret the silence that surrounds it. Someone who is experiencing the distress of a snowstorm cannot understand why you don't come to assist them and most often sees this silence as a rejection or disapproval. And then there is the awkwardness of reconnection after a prolonged period of not having had contact. How do you behave when you first meet again? Do you acknowledge what has happened? The stories of many, many people have taught me that the gap just grows bigger until it is too large to bridge, and then people simply avoid each other.

When we encounter grief and the obvious anguish of a grieving person, we naturally feel helpless. In order to diminish this feeling, people seek to alleviate the anguish of the bereft, or at least try to fix their problem. If they see an improvement, they feel they have contributed something. As a consequence they feel better. However, when responding to a grieving person we need to stay with our feeling of helplessness, and simply be with the other person, anguish and all, rather than try to alter their behaviour.

It is of course difficult to know how much to get involved. We try to find a balance between being intrusive and being respectful. In other words, what dose of ourselves do we administer? Too much of me can be an overdose, too little and I am ineffectual. And caring can also become toxic. A toxic dose is where we take over and begin to control. This is the difference between caring for someone and 'care-taking'.

For example:

It is 'care-taking' when we assume responsibility for meeting the needs of others – even those needs which they should meet without us. We care for someone when we do not do what they can and should do for themselves, and do what they truly need.

It is 'care-taking' when we expect others to live up to our expectations supposedly 'for their own good'. When we make no demands and do not become upset when their behaviour goes against our advice, then we are caring for them.

It is 'care-taking' when we feel responsible for the feelings of others and believe it is our fault if they are sad. When we care for another we recognise that our behaviour affects them but that their reaction to our behaviour produces their feelings. We are not responsible for the emotional states of others.

A most important first step in being able to respond to those who are grieving is to learn how to be with them without trying to control or influence them in what they say or do.

Learn to Show Love, Not Control

'Just let me talk. Most of the time I just need to hear out loud what is going on inside my head. I don't want your advice or to hear what you would do if you were me.'

Many of our responses are negative. We don't intend them to be, but that does not alter the effect they have on other people. They are negative because they diminish self-esteem, and decrease the likelihood that others will find their own solutions. Negative responses usually trigger defensiveness and resentment because they suggest inadequacy. They are particularly destructive because they nearly always prevent true expression. Here are a few common responses; they are unhelpful and we need to learn to avoid them.

Advice-giving

When we give unasked for advice, or tell someone else what to do, it is an insult to their intelligence. Giving advice implies a lack of confidence in their capacity to understand and cope with difficulties. In effect we are saying that 'I know better than you do', even though we are not the one who has had the loss and who is grieving. In the face of such advice-giving (which is usually delivered with utter conviction), people tend to think that their behaviour is being judged or criticised, and they then become defensive or withdraw. Another problem with advice is that the advisor seldom understands the full implications of the problem. People habitually give advice but would not recognise that they do so.

Logical argument

Logic focuses on facts and avoids feelings. In situations of personal distress logic keeps everyone at an emotional distance. When logic is used to avoid emotional involvement, you are withdrawing from the other person at a most inopportune moment, and in doing so are denying them their feelings. People then see themselves and their feelings as unacceptable.

Reassuring

Reassurance is often used by people who like the idea of being helpful, but who do not want to experience the emotional demand that goes with it. It is a way of apparently comforting someone while actually doing the opposite. Too often the reassurances are false, or they are delivered in the form of clichés, all of which tend to trivialise what has happened. Reassurance is actually a form of emotional withdrawal. They may convey sympathy – or pity – but not empathy.

Diverting

When we switch a conversation to our own topic, we are diverting away from another's concerns. Some people do this because they need to grab attention for themselves, but more commonly people resort to diversion when they are uncomfortable with the emotions stimulated by the conversation. Being with a grieving person is a sure-fire guarantee that our own stored emotions will be aroused, so diverting, deflecting or ignoring another's concerns is a common response. However, when we do divert a conversation, the message conveyed is that we don't consider the issue important.

When we use these responses, our own feelings of helplessness might be reduced and we might genuinely believe we have been able to assist the grieving person. Usually people who use these responses remain unaware of the critical judgement they have imposed or the effect of their intervention. Learn to listen to the substance of what a person is saying rather than thinking you have to give your opinion.

Another very real reason why people feel helpless and 'leave them to get over it' is because there is little other than personal experience to prepare us for loss. Inexperience and the absence of grief education make it difficult to recognise and understand the normal responses of grieving people. A first step towards rendering effective assistance is to develop your own knowledge.

Be Sure of the Facts

For each person the process of grieving is unique. We cannot expect someone to behave according to our expectations or preconceived ideas.

Many people give advice to grieving people when they have never been through a similar experience, nor had any formal instruction about grief or bereavement. I can only surmise that their expertise stems from popular myth and their own (untested) beliefs. Be aware, then, of the extent of your own knowledge before you rush to give advice and learn to recognise how your own experience (or lack of it) influences your responses. Listed below are ten key points that are addressed in this book. Be conversant with them, and adjust your expectations accordingly.

- Grieving is a natural, normal process.
- If often lasts a very long time.
- Grief is expressed and resolved differently by each person.
- The amount of grief a person experiences is usually a reflection of how important the loss is to them.
- It is hard for people to grieve when others comment on their tears, or make comments that suggest judgement, criticism or inadequacy.
- Grief is also cumulative. It means that if a previous major loss or death has not been grieved appropriately or adequately, then that old grief will add to the new grief.
- Grief can be delayed. This means that a person might not begin to grieve until a long time after a death or loss has occurred.

- Grief affects the total person and will also cause a change in behaviour.
- Grieving is a social process, and the support of others is needed to successfully complete it.
- Grief does not just go away or get better. It needs work to become resolved.

Becoming familiar with the causes, symptoms, needs and management of grief, will help you become clear about which interventions are helpful, which are not, and why. I hope you will also come to appreciate that there is no right or wrong way to grieve, and instead will consider how best to assist someone to do it their way.

The Initial Contact

The most important objective for a helper is to enable the grieving person to explore their own thoughts and feelings.

The first thing to do before making contact with a grieving person is to prepare yourself. It is realistic to expect someone to become upset when you talk about what has happened or mention the name of the person who has died. Let go of any fear or guilt that you have caused them to be upset. When you are able to do this, you are on your way, because now you can be of assistance, instead of just being 'nice'.

Be clear about your role and the purpose for your visit, or why you are making contact, as this will determine both your manner and approach. Your role may vary, e.g. health care professional, bereavement support person, friend, concerned neighbour, polite inquiring social club member. Each role suggests different responsibilities, and requires differing levels of skill and expertise.

Begin to monitor your own behaviour. Become conscious of what you say, how you say it, when you interrupt and for what reason, and eliminate unhelpful responses. This will take time and practice, but developing awareness is the first step to mastery.

We can show our interest by asking questions. Ask questions without being aggressive, and to show genuine interest. In this way you will avoid appearing nosey. If you are a stranger, I recommend you introduce yourself, where you are from, and get straight to the reason for your visit. Safety is created by your integrity which is conveyed by your respect, demeanour and genuine interest.

Questions are helpful because they allow us to express our interest. I have learnt to avoid asking too many in rapid succession (as the experience becomes that of being interrogated), and to phrase them generally or as an invitation to talk. In this way it avoids a specific focus and allows the person to answer as they choose.

Some useful starting phrases

- Tell me a little about the loss/death.

  (Gives the grieving person a clear indication that you are willing to talk about the incident, and are interested in doing so.)

- Tell me from the beginning … about him/her, the relationship.

  (Opens up the history behind what has happened and provides opportunity for review.)

- What happened that day?
  (Reveals the extent of their involvement and what may need to be done now as a consequence.)

- How have things been with you since this happened?
  (Explores family connections and the quality and extent of social support networks.)

- What does this mean to you?
  (Affords insight into the significance of the loss and possible ramifications.)

- What else is happening for you?
  (Reveals possible sources of stress.)

- Have you been through any other bad times like this?
  (Highlights previous grief situations that may not be resolved.)

These are merely suggestions for getting started and building bridges. Once you have made this effort, however stumbling, the person will respond with as much as they feel free to at that time. Your focus then is on them and what they are saying. What you then contribute will come from your listening and observations. Remember, you are not responsible for the problem, and you don't have to fix it. It is not necessary to tell your story, although if you have had a similar experience, limited disclosure may be helpful. If you do choose to share something of your own experience, be clear why you are doing so and always finish by returning the focus to the other person. Allow silence and increase your capacity to tolerate it.

- Express yourself honestly, and let your genuine concern and caring show.
- Be yourself, as you need to be comfortable with what you are doing throughout.
- Laugh, cry and be angry, but remain in control of yourself and the situation. They are in no position to be looking after you.
- Answer questions honestly and gently. Never lie. If you don't know the answer, say so, and offer to find out.
- Learn to be with the person, rather than the problem.
- Expect that they will become tired very easily. Grieving is hard work.

Assisting the grieving is not so much about 'doing' something as simply 'being' with them. In accepting people as they are, giving them permission to do as they need and supporting them throughout, you will have helped enormously. If in doubt about any intervention, express your intention and give them the opportunity to comment or decide.

Helpful Responses

Respond only to what has been asked. If people want to know more, they will ask later. Too much information too soon can feel hurtful.

Often the most meaningful communication is non-verbal. By just being there you are sharing your concern, support and love.

Learn to allow people to say what they need to tell, without expressing an opinion about what they say, or the language they use.

When offering help, be specific about what you can offer and are prepared to do. For example, say that you will provide a meal one night a week or can provide transport to the hospital in the afternoons, rather than 'If you need anything give me a ring'. *Unless of course you are prepared to do anything, at any time.*

When helping to organise activity or offering information, write it down and give it to the person. Don't just give a verbal message and expect them to remember.

Avoid putting a time limit on their grieving. It is different for everyone and it does not help when we try to define it.

Some Dos

- Acknowledge that the person's style of grieving will be unique and different from everyone else.
- Talk about the loss.
- Talk about the special endearing qualities of the person who has died.
- Try to understand the nature of the loss and its ramifications.
- Allow realistic time to grieve – remember this is a process, not an event.
- Encourage them to be patient with themselves.
- Allow people to have real memories of what has been lost – don't idealise or pacify.
- Recognise the intensity of grief that will be experienced at certain significant times (anniversaries, birthdays, Christmas).
- Encourage people to express emotion and to work through their grief.

- Remember that children grieve too and allow them to grieve with the adults.
- Give hugs and touch, where appropriate, if you are comfortable doing this.
- Affirm people and encourage them to do things for themselves.
- Allow some private time. Be there, but don't smother the person you're helping.
- Offer help, but let them decide what they are ready for.
- Help to organise immediate but simple things, e.g. keeping the mail straight, shopping, errands, make a list of things to do, note phone calls, visitors, people who bring food.

Things to be Avoided

'Please don't tell me what I should feel. And I am not interested in knowing what you would do if you were me.'

Avoid escalating comments that in any way suggest blame, revenge or which infer that the care given in hospital or by others was inadequate. The grieving are plagued by feelings of doubt and guilt without any help from their family and friends.

Don't be put off by repetitive knock-backs to your efforts to assist. Your offers will be appreciated, and it is heartening for people to know that you are still keeping in contact. Be available but undemanding. When your offers of assistance and invitations to socialise are declined, this is because it is more than the person is ready to cope with. It is not a personal rejection of you.

Avoid causing more grief by removing tasks, responsibilities or activities from the grieving person without their permission. They may wish to remain involved in things they can handle.

Avoid the urge to have a clean out or remove articles and belongings for someone. When the person is ready they will take care of this in their own way, or ask for help.

Some Don'ts

- Don't generalise their situation.
- Don't assume you know best.
- Don't prevent the grieving from expressing their guilt or anger if they need to.
- Don't stifle the grieving person's desire to talk about their loss or deceased.
- Don't say they ought to be feeling better by now or anything else which implies a judgement about their feelings or progress.
- Don't preach at them or try to find something positive, like a moral lesson, in what has happened.
- Don't keep someone busy in order to avoid the emptiness and pain of grief.
- Don't minimise, trivialise or make comparisons about the loss.
- Don't give false reassurances.
- Don't push alcohol or pills at them. If medication is necessary let a trained person provide it.

Please Don't Tell Me

'*Words aren't even necessary. Just being there, holding my hand, crying with me or listening to me would be much more comforting than the words they feel they must say.*'

'*You're the richer for having had them/it.*'
   Right now I'm bereft and the poorer for having lost it

'*You'll be reunited with them one day.*'
   My life is here and now and every moment accentuates their absence.

'*You'll understand it all one day.*'
   Promises, promises. I need an explanation now.

'*There is light at the end of the tunnel.*'
   What tunnel is that? My vision is consumed with blackness right now.

'*It's all God's will.*'
   I cannot understand how God could cause me so much despair and pain.

'*Count your blessings.*'
   I cannot in my wildest imaginings consider all this pain, this tragedy, this anger, this emptiness, to be a blessing.

'*You are now the little man, or woman, about the house.*'
   That is too much adult responsibility for me just now, and it robs me of my childhood.

   These are but some of the clichés of grief. The most common is one we have probably all uttered at some stage: 'I know how you feel'. You may honestly believe that you know how someone else is feeling. You may have been in exactly the same situation, but all you really know is what you felt at that time. Because of this you may be able to make a fairly accurate guess about what someone might be experiencing. But you can never know, and they resent the fact that you tell them you do.

Clichés like these are superficial and using them is the quickest way to dismiss someone and end a conversation. It may be years before a person can gain insight from their experience and consequently be able to count their blessings. To say something like this to a person who is in the midst of loss and grief simply conveys the message that the speaker has no appreciation of what that person is experiencing and no willingness to do so.

- Try to see things from the grieving person's point of view.
- Do be aware of the added responsibilities and changes that person now faces.

Looking After Yourself

Problems arise when our actions say one thing, and our words, another.

It's wise not to focus so much on the needs of the grief-stricken that you neglect yourself. Remain alert to your needs and be mindful that meeting these are as important as meeting the needs of the grieving. We are only able to offer as much as we give to ourselves.

Be careful not to underestimate the effect that supporting someone will have on you. You will quite naturally experience a depth and range of feelings, and be extremely tired at times. It is important to acknowledge and respect these feelings. You may need to find someone you can talk to about your experience and feelings. Don't suppress your own emotions dishonestly. Keep your own support systems nourished and use them frequently as a source of support, assurance and redirection.

As a helper, you will be affected by being involved. Supporting someone who is grieving is one experience that is guaranteed to push all your buttons. Any stored or unresolved grief that you have will surface. It is a natural part of the process and it happens to us all. But it is important to deal with what is raised for you separately, so that it will not contaminate your care-giving. Responsible health care professionals have supervision to assist with this. Rather than fall into shame or denial, enlist the guidance of a professional and deal with the issue. It is time to do so; that is why the problem has arisen now.

Be gentle with yourself. Have realistic expectations, and remember that you are but one person and a link in a chain for the grieving person. Learn to set realistic boundaries for yourself and to say 'no'. If you can never say no, what is your 'yes' worth? Recognise and accept your own limitations.

As suggested, develop your own grief knowledge so that you have a sound basis for your interventions rather than letting them come from your own feelings or making assumptions. Remember that in light of the pain you will see, you are bound to feel helpless at times, and that being there is more important than doing.

- Do something creative to recharge your batteries frequently.
- Maintain your sense of humour and learn to play.
- Learn about the signs of burn-out and when to take time out.

- Take time to think and pray. It is medicine for the mind and soothing to the soul.
- Don't try to be all things to all people.
- Abandon any need to be in control.
- Learn to be comfortable with ambiguity.

Putting It All Together

Support often means listening to the same story – again and again – many months after the event.

Our attitude is central in determining how we respond to the grieving. After you have read the information given here, I hope you will be drawn to reflect on, or change your attitude about 'leaving them to get over it'. Our attitudes and expectations affect each other, and both influence our behaviour. And our behaviour impacts on others, whether we intend it to or not.

I leave you then with a set of attitudes, or way of being, that will best assist you to help a friend in grief.

THE BE ATTITUDES
Be Aware
Remember that grief work is normal, and a necessary process.

Be There
Learn to be with the person, rather than trying to solve the problem.

Be Sensitive
Allow the pain. Don't stop it, or minimise it, or try to take it away.

Be Human

Allow expression of feelings (including guilt, anger, sorrow, and depression) without offering your opinion, or judgement.

Be Ready

To listen when the story is told over and over again.

Be Patient

Remember that the process of grieving is demanding, painful and takes time.

Food For Thought

A friend is one
to whom
one may pour out
all the contents
of one's heart,
chaff and grain together,
knowing
that the gentlest of hands
will take and sift it:
keep what is worth keeping
and with the breath of kindness
blow the rest away.

Arabian proverb

Personal Reflection

When responding to a grieving person:

Do encourage the person to talk

 Do not ....

Do help them identify their support system

 Do not ....

Do present a realistic picture of grief

 Do not ....

Do allow people to deal with their grief as they want to

 Do not ....

Do focus on the person and their loss and their grief

 Do not ....

Do be aware of what is happening for you

 Do not ....

Do try and see the loss and grief from the other person's point of view

 Do not ....

Do avoid platitudes and euphemisms

 Do not ....

Do accept the grieving person without criticism or judgement

 Do not ....

Do be specific about how, or if, you can be of help

 Do not ....

Do let your genuine concern and caring show

 Do not ....

Summary of Key Points

- Leaving someone to get over it alone adds pain to an already intolerably painful experience.

- In light of the pain and distress you will see, it is natural to feel helpless.

- When responding to a grieving person, we need to learn to increase our ability to stay with our own feelings of helplessness.

- You are not responsible for anyone else's pain. Neither is it your responsibility to solve the problem.

- There is a big difference between caring for someone and 'care-taking'.

- Learn to show love rather than control.

- Ensure the accuracy of any information you offer.

- Avoid using euphemisms and giving false reassurances.

- Remain alert to your own needs and be mindful that meeting them is as important as meeting the needs of the person you are supporting.

conclusion

I suspect after reading this, life will never be quite the same again. At the very least, you will never be able to quote one of the myths I have addressed without pausing to think. At best, I hope this material will make a difference to the way you reflect on your own history, and in the way you approach people who have experienced various kinds of dramatic loss.

My hunch is that you will now find yourself faced with having to make a choice. Do you accept what I have said? If so, you will assume responsibility for, and attend to, your own unresolved grief. Or do you dismiss my writing as interesting, but irrelevant? If so, you can continue life as before.

Be mindful that in making this decision, others will be affected by your choice. The effects of unresolved grief are passed from generation to generation, as is the model of healthy grief work. Receptive, impressionable, young minds will notice and learn from you and what you do. Those to whom this book is dedicated are an example: each has grief to face as the result of the unresolved issues of a previous generation.

There are many more myths that are used in response to grief, but now I hope you will pause long enough to question the validity and sincerity of anything that is said before taking it on board or offering it to others.

To those of you who have already revisited and begun to rethink your emotional territory, I sincerely hope you find this work informative and helpful. I know the process will not be an easy one for you, but take courage: it is the road to becoming fully alive.

selected bibliography

David Adams and Eleanor Deveau (eds), *Beyond the Innocence of Childhood, Volume 3: Helping Children and Adolescents Cope with Death and Bereavement* (New York: Baywood, 1995)

Ellen Bass and Laura Davis, *The Courage to Heal* (New York: Harper & Row, 1988)

Melody Beattie, *Codependents' Guide to the Twelve Steps* (New York: Bantam, 1992)

Andrew Bell, *Creative Control* (Auckland: Tandem, 1994)

Rusty Berkus, *To Heal Again: Towards serenity and the resolution of grief.* (California: Red Rose, 1984)

Claudia Black, *It's Never Too Late to Have a Happy Childhood* (New York: Ballantine, 1989)

Robert Bolton, *People Skills* (Australia: Simon & Schuster, 1987)

John Bowlby, *Attachment and Loss, Voume 1: Attachment* (London: Hogarth, 1969)

John Bowlby, *Attachment and Loss, Volume 2: Separation: Anxiety and Anger* (London: Hogarth, 1979)

John Bowlby, *Attachment and Loss, Volume 3: Loss* (London: Hogarth, 1980)

John Bowlby, *The Making and Breaking of Affectional Bonds* (London: Tavistock, 1979)

Gene Combs and Jill Freedman, *Symbol, Story and Ceremony* (New York: Norton, 1990)

Study Course; Death and Bereavement Educational Services (Victoria: 1983)

Merle Fossum and Marilyn Mason, *Facing Shame* (New York: Norton, 1986)

Robert Fulton and others (eds), *Death and Dying, Challenge and Change* (California: Addison-Wesley, 1978)

Geoffrey T. Glassock and Louise Rowling, *Learning to Grieve* (Newtown: Millennium, 1992)

Graeme Griffin and Des Tobin, *In the Midst of Life: The Australian Response to Death* (Melbourne: University Press, 1982)

Earle Grollman, *Suicide: Prevention, Intervention, Postvention* (Boston: Beacon Press, 1988)

Robin Haig, *The Anatomy of Grief: Biopsychosocial and Therapeutic Perspectives* (Illinois: Charles C Thomas, 1990)

John Harvey (ed), *Perspectives on Loss* (London: Taylor and Francis, 1998)

Donald Irish, Kathleen Lundquist, and Vivian Nelsen (eds), *Ethnic Variations in Dying, Death, and Grief: Diversity in Universality* (Washington: Taylor & Francis, 1993)

Lee Jampolsky, *Healing the Addictive Mind* (California: Celestial Arts, 1991)

Robert Kastenbaum, *Death, Society, and Human Experience* (New York: Macmillan, 1991)

Anne Katherine, *Boundaries* (New York: Fireside Parkside, 1991)

David Kissane and Sidney Bloch, 'Family Grief' British Journal of Psychiatry (1994) pp. 164, 728–740

Clive S. Lewis, *A Grief Observed* (London: Faber, 1961)

Janice Lord, *No Time for Goodbyes: Coping with Sorrow, Anger and Injustice after a Tragic Death* (California: Pathfinder, 1990)

Richard Loretto, *Children's Conceptions of Death* (New York: Springer, 1980)

Francis MacNab, *Life after Loss: Getting over Grief, Getting on with Life* (Philadelphia: Millennium Books, 1989)

Terry Martin and Kenneth Doka, *Men Don't Cry ... Women Do: Transcending Gender Stereotypes of Grief* (Philadelphia: Taylor and Francis, 2000)

Abraham Maslow, *Motivation and Personality* (New York: Harper and Row, 1954)

Mary Ann Morgan and John Morgan (eds), *Thanatology: A Liberal Arts Approach* (Ontario: King's College, 1988)

Caroline Myss, *Anatomy of the Spirit: The Seven Stages of Power and Healing* (New York: Bantam Books, 1996)

Jules Older, *Touching is Healing* (New York: Stein and Day, 1985)

Merren Parker, *A Time to Grieve* (Auckland: Methuen, 1981)

Colin M. Parkes, *Bereavement: Studies of Grief in Adult Life* (Middlesex: Penguin, 1972)

Therese Rando, *Treatment of Complicated Mourning* (Illinois: Research, 1993)

Beverley Raphael, *The Anatomy of Bereavement: A Handbook for the Caring Professions* (London: Unwin Hyman, 1984)

Linford Rees, *A New Short Textbook of Psychiatry* (London: Hodder and Stoughton, 1988)

Carl Rogers, *On Becoming a Person* (London: Constable, 1982)

Virginia Satir, *Self Esteem* (California: Celestial Arts, 1975)

Anne Wilson Schaef, *Co-Dependence, Misunderstood-Mistreated* (San Francisco: Harper, 1986)

Carol Staudacher, *Beyond Grief: A Guide for Recovering from the Death of a Loved One* (Oakland: New Harbinger, 1987)

Scott Sullender, *Grief and Growth: Pastoral Resources for Emotional and Spiritual Growth* (New York: Paulist Press, 1960)

Ann Stearns, *Coming Back: Rebuilding Lives After Crisis and Loss* (London: Cedar, 1988)

Sue Patton Thoele, *The Courage to be Yourself* (Nevada City: Pyramid, 1988)

Barbara Ward, *Healing Grief* (London: Vermilion, 1993)

Hannelore Wass and Robert Neimeyer (eds), *Dying: Facing the Facts* (London: Taylor and Francis, 1998)

William Worden, *Grief Counselling and Grief Therapy: A handbook for the mental health practitioner.* (New York: Springer, 1982)

Irvin D. Yalom, *Existential Psychotherapy* (New York: Basic Books, 1980)

finding grief support

The following list offers an overview of where to obtain information about resources and services for grief support.

Note that what is available will vary from region to region.

The fact that an organisation is included is not a personal endorsement of its healthy operation. Please refer to guidelines mentioned in Chapter 8 regarding support groups.

For Local Support Information

Look in your Yellow Pages for:

Citizens Advice Bureau

Offers a confidential telephone service, face-to-face interview, or advice on consumer matters to anyone needing help or advice, or seeking information on resources within the community. Referral and assistance to find the best agency for particular needs.

Lifeline

Offers skilled listeners through a confidential telephone service at times of crisis. Will have information about local agencies and resources.

Youthline

Free and confidential telephone listening, information and referral service, mainly for young people, but available for all. Will have information about local agencies and resources.

City/Town Council

Check with the individual or department responsible for Social Services. Most will have a directory of community and social services information. It will include a comprehensive list of Health and Disability Groups in your district, contact details, and the services they offer.

For Specialist Support

The National Association for Loss And Grief (NZ) Ltd (NALAG)

NALAG's main aim is to encourage and promote professional and community education in the process and consequences of loss and grief. A wide cross-section of the caring professions is represented in the NALAG membership. NALAG is aware of the network of support and resources in the community and can often make useful suggestions when assistance is required.

Contact Details: National Administrator
                        P.O. Box 674
                        Napier
                        Fax 06 843 9365

Skylight

A national organisation working to support children, young people and their families who have been affected by change, loss and grief. Skylight provides:

- education and training for those who work with and care for grieving children and young people, and their families
- a national resource and information service on issues of loss and grief
- a counselling/support service for children, young people and their families
- advocacy to enhance understanding of, and services for, grieving families

Skylight's head office is in Wellington but it also has branch offices in Christchurch and Auckland.

Contact Details: 0800 299 100
                        Fax: 04 939 4759
                        P.O. Box 7309
                        Wellington South
                        Email: info@skylight-trust.org.nz

Funeral Directors

Many firms now offer bereavement support services, although what they offer varies greatly. Services may include a library service, home visits, phone support, and grief support groups. Support services may be offered routinely to people who have used the company at the time of a death, but some directors now make their support groups available to the public on a fee paying basis.

Hospice

Hospices provide bereavement support for those family members who have been involved with their programme. The range of support varies, but many hospices now include professional counselling services and grief support groups. These services may be restricted to hospice clientele, but check to see what local centres offer to the public, or on a fee paying basis.

Hospital

Some hospitals offer specialist support groups through their mental health services. Some support groups may be specialised, as in Dunedin for example, where a support group for children between the ages of five and 12 years is run according to demand.

Contact Details: B.Ks Group (Bereaved Kids)
                    Paediatric Outpatients
                    Dunedin Hospital
                    Phone 03474 7975

Cancer Society

Most branches offer a variety of programmes that are designed to assist patients and carers to live with cancer. Some also offer bereavement support and/or grief counselling.

Examples of Bereavement Support Groups

Widows and Widowers Association

Social and support club for widowed people.

Baby Bereavement Group

Support for parents who have suffered the loss of a baby at any time from conception onwards.

Sudden Infant Death Syndrome (SIDS) or Cot Death Society
Support for bereaved parents who have infants die of cot death.

Compassionate Friends
Support group for bereaved parents whose child has died at any age, by whatever means.

Bereaved by Suicide
Support for those affected by the suicide of a loved one.

Other Avenues of Assistance

Counselling Services
Many people go to a counsellor who has been recommended to them by a friend. You can also find a counsellor by checking in the Yellow Pages. Look under Counselling Services, Psychotherapists and Psychotherapy Services. Choosing a counsellor who has professional qualifications ensures that they are trained and that the quality of their work and service is regularly monitored. When a counsellor is a member of a professional association, it means that they are accountable to that association and its supervisory procedures, and that you will be protected by that Association's Code of Ethics and Complaints Procedure. Request an initial interview and then ask yourself if you feel you could be open with this person, and if you feel understood by them. Proceed on the basis of how you answer these questions.

Workplace Chaplaincy Services
Qualified chaplains and counsellors provide personal and organisa tional support to people and their work places.

Church Agencies
Many provide a range of services for families and individuals which include professional counselling, education programmes, family support and community programmes.

Victim Support

A 24-hour service for people who are victims of crimes, fire or accidents. Offers practical support, advice and advocacy that is free and confidential. Does not offer counselling services.

Library Services

Most libraries will have some reading material on grief. Check to see how it has been catalogued. Key words under which to search include grief, death, bereavement, psychology, thanatology.

Websites

The Internet can provide general information on grief as well as access to many support groups.